ƒP

Stop Your Cravings

A Balanced Approach
to Burning Fat, Increasing Energy,
and Reducing Stress

JENNIFER WORKMAN, M.S., R.D.

The Free Press

NEW YORK   LONDON   TORONTO   SYDNEY   SINGAPORE

THE FREE PRESS
A division of Simon & Schuster, Inc.
1230 Avenue of the Americas
New York, NY 10020

For information about special discounts for bulk purchases,
please contact Simon & Schuster Special Sales:
1-800-456-6798 or business@simonandschuster.com

Designed by Stratford Publishing

Manufactured in the United States of America

1   3   5   7   9   10   8   6   4   2

Library of Congress Cataloging-in-Publication Data

Workman, Jennifer, 1965–
Stop your cravings : a balanced approach to burning fat,
increasing energy, and reducing stress / Jennifer Workman.
p.   cm.
Includes bibliographical references and index.
1. Nutrition.   2. Health.   3. Weight loss.
4. Medicine, Ayurvedic.   I. Title.
RA784 .W76   2002
613.7—dc21   2001040893

ISBN 0-7432-1705-5 (alk. paper)

Dedication

I have been blessed with many wonderful people in my life, some for too short a time. It has made me question: Why am I here, how long am I here for, and what am I supposed to do with the time I have?

The answers have become very clear in the more than two and a half years I have worked on this project. I am here to live life to the fullest, to never forget to tell the people I love that I love them, and to thank my angels for every lesson and teacher that crosses my path.

I would like to dedicate this book to all the special people who have come and gone, but especially to Janine Crocitto and to my grandmother Ida Workman. It was because of the two of them that I started searching for new answers. And to all the children who go to bed without enough food, alone and hungry. I hope to make a bit of difference and leave the world a little more aware and kind and gentle. They have truly guided this project.

Contents

Part Two
A Simple Action Plan

Acknowledgments

I can never thank my family enough for all their help and support. To my parents, Pat and Stan Workman: I love you both so very much, and thank you for believing in me. I would not have been able to do this without you. You have given me strength and inspired me never to settle, never to give up, to stand up for the underdog, to appreciate simplicity, and to see the beauty in the world, even when it's not so beautiful. I am very lucky to have you for my parents.

My thanks also go:

To my brothers, Keith and Michael, who have also learned many lessons about love and loss, but who have remained good, kind, strong, amazing souls, always there for their friends and family. Thank you both for all your support.

To my aunt Julie, a gentle soul who would like to see the world be a bit more kind and compassionate. And to my sister-in-law, Sandy, another gentle person who would like to change the world. To her wonderful family in New York and Ecuador, who give from their hearts and always remind me that you don't need to have a lot to love and laugh. To my Workman, Goldstein, and Mooney families, too; family, food, laughter, and love have *always* been their first priorities. Thank you all for your support and enthusiasm.

To my clients, who have asked for help and have taken a chance on something new and different. I appreciate your search for new answers and trust in the process.

To Sarasvati Buhrman, my teacher and friend for the past five years. She has helped me to see the world in a better way, with more clarity and insight, and she has given me the tools to learn how to stay balanced and to get through life when it isn't so easy.

To Pat Hansen, another amazing woman who has graced this world with her strength, love, compassion, and wisdom, for living your message and giving the rest of us an incredible example to follow. And Dr. Vasant Lad, who has given me permission to attempt to take some of his experience and wisdom and try to help America find nurturance and balance.

To Gigia Kolouch, what can I say? She has worked with me on this project for more than four years, believing in the mission even when we had no money and no time. Her energy and love and passion for food, children, the planet, art, and flowers are evident in this book. It has been an honor working with her.

To Karen Bucklin, my right hand (and my left). An angel who showed up just at the right time to manage the business and help us continue to move forward. She has believed in our project and has been willing to back up her belief with her time and energy and love. She is another spirit who sees the world for what it could be—gentle and more compassionate.

To Ben Velàzquez and his family. He has been my friend for more than fourteen years. We have seen too many of the not-so-nice parts of life together, yet he has remained a strong and true friend, with a great heart and great vision. He is always there for his family and friends. This book is also dedicated to his dad, Stan, and his brother, Sam, who have also guided me on this project.

To Oatmeal and Berri, my furry family, and Amber Adkerson, a beautiful golden child sent to me by the universe so that I would remember to see the magic everywhere, read more fairy tales, and laugh more.

To all the rest of my friends and coworkers in New York and Colorado, especially Jeff Bartels, Sheila Compton, and Ruthie Papavassilio, my Colorado family, true spirits who have graced my life with love and laughter and spirit I didn't even know existed until I met them.

To Indira and Vijay Gupta, who have added love and laughter and positive energy to this project. Indira's spirit and voice are always enough to get me motivated and inspired to keep going. Her love and energy are in this book too.

To all the brilliant chefs who so generously contributed their recipes. They are truly dedicated to creating a better environment and work very hard to offer safe, healthy, and incredibly wonderful food.

To Christine Caldwell, Denny Thompson, Trace Westlake, Barbara Biziou, Pamela Serure, Charles Poliquin, Don Bruce, Billy Corbett, Brian Barkley, Bobbie Nigro, Theresa Robertson, Glenn Streeter, David Sawyer, Dr. Sarita Shrestha, Leslie Kalichman, Michael Dick, John Douillard, Elaine Boudoris, Tracey Brummett, Jim Procknow, Susan Brienza, Laurelyn Baker, Caren Griffen, Jessica Dyson, Lena Falin, and all the other teachers and angels who have been there just when I needed them. They have all believed in this project and helped keep it moving forward.

To Felicia Tomasko, a wonderful friend, yoga instructor, and medical researcher who got here just in the nick of time. And Donna Romberger, illustrator, and her son, Jed, two incredible artists who added more beautiful energy to the project.

To Eileen Cope of Lowenstein Associates, Inc., an amazing literary agent, who has had the patience to walk me through all the steps it took to get this project to completion, even when my lack of experience got in the way. She has been a true motivator, believed in the higher good, and helped me keep it together. She never got tired of my questions and ignorance. This is her work as well; I greatly appreciated her patience and expertise.

To Judy Kern, an incredible writer who has also had unlimited patience, perseverance, and vision. I can't even begin to say thank you for all the time and hours we spent together. Her wisdom about the industry has been a great asset and has helped me stay grounded. She has been a great guide.

To Philip Rappaport, my editor, who has great vision and heart and was willing to see and honor the bigger picture in this project. He has been sincere and dedicated to the higher good since we met, and I appreciate his willingness to take a chance on me. Business and heart are not separate issues for Philip.

Finally, to all the other friends, family, and wonderful people— grownups and children—both here and in spirit, who have graced my life and brought me the messages I needed to hear.

INTRODUCTION

East Meets West

The Best of Both Worlds

If you're reading this book, it's probably because you already have four or five diet books on your shelf, you've tried them all, and none has worked for you over the long haul. Either you didn't lose the weight the book promised you would or the food you were "allowed" to eat was so restrictive and boring that eventually, sooner or later, you simply couldn't stick to the plan. Many of those books probably contain good, accurate, useful information. The problem, as I've discovered during my seventeen years working in the health and fitness industry, is that there's now so much information available, and so much of it appears to be contradictory, that everyone— from competitive athletes to doctors to weekend warriors to couch potatoes—is confused and frustrated.

The weight-loss industry—including diet books, diet plans, diet pills, and diet supplements—is now a $50 billion industry in the United States, yet more than 50 percent of Americans remain overweight. According to the most recent National Health and Nutrition Examination Survey, 26 percent of those are considered obese or grossly overweight, a figure that has nearly doubled in the last two decades. We're bombarded daily with nutritional information, most of us think we know what we "should" or "shouldn't" be eating, yet nothing, so far, has worked for the average American who steps on and off the diet merry-go-round three to four times each year.

A "nutraceutical" is defined as any food or part of a food that has a medical or health benefit—from dietary supplements to herbal products to processed foods. *Nutraceuticals World,* the trade magazine of the nutraceutical industry, noted in 1999 that "nine out of ten shoppers (90%) understand the relationship between nutrition and health. In fact, more than half of primary shoppers feel that just eating healthfully can greatly reduce the risk of developing certain diseases." If that's the case, there is still a piece missing from this puzzle, because we're more overweight than ever yet our diets are lacking in many nutrients, including the good, monounsaturated fats and essential fatty acids. We suffer from an overabundance of poor-quality food and a lack of activity despite the billions spent on health club memberships, exercise equipment, and personal trainers. The big question, obviously, is why, despite our apparent understanding of the issues, can virtually no one stick to a diet or an exercise plan. Why is it that, whatever the diet—whether it be for health or fitness or weight loss—Americans simply are not complying, even though we all think we know what we're "supposed" to be eating? Why are we the most diet-crazed country in the world and yet also the most overweight, and apparently the most frustrated by our failure?

My experience has shown me that the answer lies, at least in part, with our cravings for foods we think we shouldn't be eating. As soon as we become stressed or overwhelmed, those cravings take over and we "blow" our diet. We're all living with enormous amounts of stress, and those cravings are our way of trying to get some relief. But *why* do we crave what we do? And why is it that a food like chocolate can have so much power over us? I have found that the combination of Eastern medical practices, such as Ayurveda, with the modern science of Western nutrition, finally provides the answers to these continually frustrating questions.

Even so mainstream an organization as The American Dietetic Association, in a recent journal article, states that traditional approaches to weight loss simply haven't worked. "For many years, research and practice in the field of weight management has been based largely on a unidimensional, simplistic, weight-loss paradigm. The long-term success rate for persons using this paradigm has been low . . . the literature indicates that few dieters actually reach their goal weight. . . . Very few of those who do lose weight sustain their new weight; thus, they increase their risk for the development of a pattern of weight cycling." The "experts" are frustrated too.

The fact is that there is no one magic formula to satisfy everyone's individual nutritional needs. Only by satisfying our individual needs on a daily basis, as part of our everyday lifestyle, will we be able to stop the cravings that have, so far, prevented us from maintaining optimum weight and optimum health. Only Ayurveda takes into account all aspects of our physical and emotional individuality and offers a comprehensive program for daily living that allows each one of us to recognize the foods we crave as something our body needs (in a nonaddictive situation) and that we are—fruitlessly—denying. To quote one of my teachers, Pat Hansen, M.S., a co-founder of the Rocky Mountain Institute for Yoga and Ayurveda, in Boulder, Colorado: "Only Ayurveda asks the key nutritional questions—for whom? under what conditions? at what time of year?" Once you understand how to answer those questions for yourself, you will find yourself eating the foods that are appropriate to your specific physical and emotional type, under particular environmental and emotional circumstances, as dictated by the changing seasons. You'll understand how to nurture and nourish your body's needs in ways that are satisfying and healthy, by incorporating herbs and spices in simple ways that will help satisfy your taste buds, improve your digestion and energy, and even help to cut body fat, without adding additional calories, carbohydrates, or fat.

But how are you supposed to decipher all the weight loss and nutritional information that's available when even with a master's degree in nutrition and exercise physiology, and seventeen years in the fitness industry, I too have struggled with my weight and obsessed about everything I ate, as have so many other fitness and medical professionals? Although I've never been severely overweight, and I've always been active and fit, my weight has fluctuated from a low of 115 to a high of 157 pounds. Food was always an issue for me, just as it was for everyone else I knew; I was always either "watching it" or on a diet. I also suffered from digestive problems I thought were normal, and my energy and moods would fluctuate, depending on what I'd been eating. I sensed there had to be a connection, but I was as frustrated as everyone else about how to fix it, and I tried every diet out there.

Over the last five or six years, after discovering Ayurveda and "integrative" medicine, I've come to realize that food *should not* be an issue; it should help you manage stress, not create more, and food cravings are a signal that something is wrong, either physically or emotionally, and your body is trying to bring the problem to your attention. But it's been a long road to enlightenment.

When I received my undergraduate degree in nutrition and business from Queens College in 1982, fitness was not the flourishing industry it has since become. While I was still an undergraduate—actually starting when I was in high school—I had begun teaching aerobics and strength training at a well-known East Coast fitness center. I was seventeen years old, in great shape, and I loved the fitness business. I tried other fields, but I never felt I belonged in "corporate America." Helping overstressed executives get out of the office and into the gym made me happy. I then began dating a competitive natural (steroid-free) bodybuilder, learned a lot about strength training and sports nutrition, and started working toward my master's degree in nutrition and exercise physiology at New York University. As part of my coursework, I was required to complete a year's medical internship working as a clinical nutritionist with patients at Beth Israel Hospital in Manhattan. It was an eye-opening experience. All the interns at the hospital were, of course, young, and a lot of them were good-looking, but they were almost all overweight, they smoked, drank too much coffee to stay awake, didn't have time to exercise, and never got enough sleep. The people I'd met in the fitness industry weren't all perfect examples of a healthy lifestyle, but their lives revolved around health and fitness, and at the time, they appeared to be light-years ahead of the medical profession when it came to diet, exercise, and preventative health. Ironically, Beth Israel Hospital in New York City has opened an "integrative" medical division run by many prestigious medical doctors who understand the benefits of bringing both worlds together.

That year of internship cemented my determination to direct my skills in the areas of nutrition and fitness toward preventative health and teaching basic stress management and lifestyle modification. As I now explain to my clients, Western medicine is at its most brilliant in emergency situations, but the goal should be to try to avoid those emergencies.

In 1991 I accepted the position of sales and marketing director at the then brand-new Peninsula Hotel/Spa—the first day spa of its kind to open in New York City. Our clients were the high-stress, high-energy, top executives and CEOs from many of the Fortune 500 companies in midtown Manhattan. It was a great learning experience to see them rush in like madpeople and leave ninety minutes later, after a massage, or a workout, or a yoga class, purring like pussycats—more focused, centered, and grounded. During my five years at the Peninsula, I gained enormous insight into the benefits obtained by combining stress management and fitness—something that many Eastern and European cultures have known for centuries. The International Spa Association has been trying to educate Americans about the health benefits of stress management for years. Many studies show that modalities such as massage, yoga, aromatherapy, meditation, and other such techniques are not mere indulgences but preventative medicine. In the late eighties and early nineties, all this was very new. "No pain, no gain" was still the prevailing mantra of fitness enthusiasts. Now yoga, meditation, visualization, and Pilates are a common part of the fitness world.

I had also just begun to implement the nutrition program at The Peninsula and had started to introduce the concept to many of the editors of health and fitness magazines. Although it was clear the program would be successful, I knew in my heart that something was still missing—I just didn't know, at the time, what it was. We had all the information about sports nutrition, stress management, and fitness, but our clients still couldn't seem to get off the diet merry-go-round.

It was in 1994 that all the information started to come together. When I was working at the Peninsula I had the unfortunate but serendipitous experience of "blowing out" the anterior cruciate ligament (ACL) in my knee while skiing. Because I had been working out for so long, my legs were very strong but also very tight. After the accident, I had difficulty getting back my full range of motion, and physical therapy was extremely painful. Up to that point, I'd had no desire to try yoga or felt I needed any kind of stress management because, as a typical type A New Yorker, I had always considered such nonstrenuous exercise a waste of time when I could be *really* working out. I, too, belonged to the "no pain, no gain" school of fitness. Eventually, upon the urging of one of the Peninsula's yoga instructors, and against the advice of my orthopedic surgeon, who was simply unfamiliar with the therapeutic benefits of yoga, I did finally wind up in a yoga class for the injured and elderly at the Integral Yoga Center, simply because I couldn't stand the physical therapy any longer. I was amazed by the difference it made in a very short time. Although it was very gentle, it was also extremely effective. My physical therapy was no longer so torturous, and my range of motion came back much more quickly. The effect on my mind was dramatic as well, and I began to understand the benefits of "calming down" my driven personality. I can actually remember hobbling out of my first or second class and realizing that even though I was standing in the middle of Broadway, I simply didn't hear the traffic noise. I just "floated" home. It's amazing to me now to see how we all receive the lessons we need in life, even if we don't recognize them in the moment!

A lot happened that year. At about the same time, my very dear, twenty-eight-year-old friend Janine was diagnosed with leukemia, and a while later, my grandmother fell and broke her hip. For three years, my friend fought valiantly through two bone marrow transplants and three rounds of chemotherapy. Although her doctors tried their best, her body continued to deteriorate, and the treatments were very difficult for her to endure. In the end, when there was nothing left for the doctors to do, she and her family sought out a nutritionist who specialized in a holistic approach to cancer. I watched her energy and color begin to improve a bit as he attempted to help rebuild and "detoxify" her system using organic fruits and vegetables and herbs. It became a proactive experience and something positive she and her family could participate in after all the treatments. She also began to work with the yoga teacher and reiki instructor who had helped me to rehabilitate my knee. I watched Janine gain some peace spiritually, and even her physician noted that he had never before seen a patient manage pain so well at that end stage of leukemia. Even though Janine did finally pass away, it was a very sad but profound experience. It helped me to understand the power and benefits of a more "holistic" approach to life and death and of treating the "whole" person. My grandmother died three months after Janine, and I wish she had been able to receive the same kind of help, but she was never offered these complementary therapies. Her treatment followed strictly traditional, old school paradigms, and as frustrated as I was, I simply had to let her go.

After my experiences with my friend, my grandmother, and my knee, I decided it was time for me to leave the spa and fitness world and return to the medical community, but this time I wanted to be in a place that combined Eastern and Western medicine. It was in 1996 that I moved to Colorado and found work in a newly opened medical center in Denver where they were doing just that. The facility combined traditional and complementary medicine, and seeing how the two could work together was another enlightening experience. I was convinced this was the direction in which the health industry ought to be moving.

At the same time, I began working as a nutritionist with Wild Oats natural markets, where I got an astounding on-the-job education in herbal and natural medicine. It was the perfect complement to my work at the medical center. Then I met Sarasvati Buhrman, Ph.D., who holds a doctorate in anthropology and is a skilled Ayurvedic practitioner and herbalist. She is, with Pat Hansen, co-founder of the Rocky Mountain Institute for Yoga and Ayurveda in Boulder, Colorado. I wanted to learn more about yoga and meditation, and when Sarasvati found out I was a nutritionist, she suggested I take a class she was teaching in Ayurvedic medicine for Westerners. That class changed my life and my career. I finally saw the vital connections between the medical profession, the food and nutrition industries, the fitness industry, and the spa industry. Ayurveda provided the key that allowed me to understand why so many Americans were having so much trouble with weight management, digestive disorders, and the many chronic, nagging complaints that were sapping their energies and keeping them from feeling really good. And it provided me with insights into how food cravings were undermining people's attempts to comply with any dietary regimen they might try. The answers were there. Why hadn't I ever heard of this before, even though I had worked in the industry so long and held a master's degree in nutrition?

Many Eastern medical practices, such as acupuncture, which stems from traditional Chinese medicine, have gained a degree of acceptance in the United States and are now approved by the Food and Drug Administration (FDA). Yoga and Ayurveda, however, are just beginning to gain a degree of generalized popularity or understanding in this country. I think one of the reasons it's been a slow integration is because these Eastern practices seem so vast and "foreign" to the typical American that simply the thought of attempting to master their intricacies is too daunting for most people. And even those who have heard about it might think that following an Ayurvedic diet would mean eating nothing but Indian food.

I believe that we have found a way to make a few of the basic principles of Ayurveda a bit simpler and easier to understand, and more applicable to the traditional Western lifestyle. My business, The Balanced Approach, started growing as I began to learn how to help clients incorporate basic Ayurvedic principles into a simple day-to-day routine. Bringing the wisdom of the East to the people of the West has become my dharma, or life's work, as they say in Eastern philosophy. I hope that by doing so, I will help you find peace with the food you eat; improve your energy level, your digestion, and your health; and, at the same time, attain the degree of fitness and the weight you have always been seeking. The fun part is learning about taste and spices and flavors to help you feel satisfied and reach your goals.

Ayurveda is a five-thousand-year-old medical healing system that originates from India but whose principles can be applied to meet the needs of any individual of any cultural background. To quote from the *International Journal of Integrative Medicine,* it is "one of the oldest forms of medicine in the world, and the forerunner of other great systems of medicine. It is one of five government-approved medical models in present-day India, and is also recognized by the World Health Organization as a viable system of natural medicine." The word *Ayurveda* translates to mean "the science of life." Its theories will complement any health, medical, or fitness program and hold true whether you're eating in a salad bar on Fifth Avenue, in a Japanese or Mexican restaurant, or in a kitchen in Des Moines. It provides insights into how to understand your individual genetic constitutional type, how to listen to your body to determine its responses to stress, foods, weather changes, and other internal and external conditions that can cause your system to go out of balance, and how to learn when it is necessary to change or moderate your diet in order to adjust to your own changing physical and emotional needs. It is a gentle and nurturing medical system that can work in conjunction with Western medicine and sports nutrition to individualize virtually any fitness program or medical treatment plan.

Western medicine is based on a knowledge of biochemistry and macronutrients—the correct ratios of proteins, fats, and carbohydrates—but, as I've discovered in the course of my seventeen-year journey (and as more and more people are now beginning to understand), Western medicine doesn't have all the answers. Even doctors who are skilled in complementary medicine, whether they are naturopaths, osteopaths, or M.D.'s, I find, are still missing some valuable information about their clients if they aren't familiar with the concept of differing constitutional types and the ways each is affected by stress and the environment. By mastering the basic principles of Ayurveda, you can come to understand the "qualities" of food—such as whether they are light or heavy, dry or oily, hot or cold—how they apply to what you eat day to day, and how they correlate to your cravings. We'll be discussing these qualities in detail in the following chapter; suffice it to say here that the concept explains how the various nutrients work with your own body to keep your systems in balance and working as efficiently as possible—and it allows you to understand why, on a hot summer day, you are likely to crave something creamy, cold, and sweet, such as a mocha frappaccino.

But this is not an either/or situation. I certainly haven't forgotten about or cast aside everything I'd previously learned about nutrition and biochemistry. Rather, I've found that what I've learned from Ayurveda works as a perfect complement to Western medicine and Western nutrition or to any other philosophy. It provides the perfect *balanced approach* to nutritional health and fitness.

Personally, I've finally arrived at a place where I'm at peace with food, and I'm happy to say that many of my clients are getting there, too. Maintaining my weight is no longer a problem; it's not something I even have to think about anymore, and I'm *never* "on a diet." I know from my own experience that it's possible to create strong digestion, lose body fat, increase energy, look younger, feel stronger, and still eat food that is satisfying, sensual, nurturing, and nourishing. But how could you, as a layperson, be expected to figure it out if so many of the experts are as frustrated in their efforts to solve the health and weight problems in this country as you are?

My goal is to help people who are frustrated about food and dieting to understand these principles. I believe my job as a nutritionist is to bring together the incredible wealth of information available from all sources—Ayurveda, the Western medical profession, the fitness industry, and Western and integrative nutritional science—and try to explain it in a way that is practical, simple, and applicable to a hectic, busy lifestyle. I would also like to help Americans realize that, above all, food should be pleasurable. In fact, you might say that my real goal is to help re-create the entire nutritional paradigm in America!

Unfortunately, most Americans have come to think of food as the enemy, when in fact it is the giver of life. We're phobic about fat, and most of us simply don't get enough protein. We seem to think that satisfying our hunger is "giving in" to weakness, and the notion that we ought to derive sensory satisfaction from food has all but flown out the window. In *Stop Your Cravings* I'll be offering many suggestions and recipes for ways to combine different tastes, textures, and qualities of food, and I'll explain how to use herbs and spices in ways that are simple but satisfying. I'll include simple recipes from chefs and cooking instructors who will show you how truly easy this can be. Too many Americans have lost touch with what it's like to cook and eat whole fresh foods—foods that really do taste much better and actually take less time to prepare because their natural flavors are so much more vibrant and distinctive. I'll even take you on a shopping trip through the supermarket and health food store, aisle by aisle, so that you'll always have a pantry full of the ingredients you need to create simple meals that you'll *like*, meals that are appropriate for your particular constitutional type, meals that will keep your body in balance and your weight where you want it to be. My goal is to help you build muscle, trim fat, and become grounded and balanced—an energized, lean, mean fighting machine.

Do you like Italian food? Mexican food? Chinese or Japanese food? Have you been taught to believe that Italian has too much pasta, Mexican and Chinese have too much fat, and Japanese has too much salt? Nothing could be further from the truth. In fact, these traditional "ethnic" cuisines actually provide a much better way of eating than the starchy, carbohydrate-heavy, low-fat diet most Americans have been following in an effort to stay slim and healthy—an effort, by the way, that has obviously failed to achieve its purpose. The traditional Mediterranean, Asian, Indian, and Mexican diets are based on a balance of good protein, healthy fats and oils, and non-gluten carbohydrates, flavored with aromatic herbs and spices to provide a variety of satisfying tastes that also strengthen and maximize digestion and health.

I arrived at The Balanced Approach as the name for my nutrition/weight management program because I think it so clearly encompasses the various aspects of what I am trying to convey. It refers to integrating a balance between the ancient wisdom of Ayurveda and the modern wisdom of Western nutritional science. It reflects the idea that once you learn how to keep your body in balance, you will begin to digest and utilize the foods you eat with greater efficiency. And it underscores the importance of achieving a proper balance among the proteins, fats, and carbohydrates that are appropriate for your particular constitutional type and your exercise or activity level.

Once you understand these basic principles and begin to apply them, you'll be surprised by how much better you feel, you'll wonder at the variety of discomforts you used to think of as "normal," and you'll be thrilled as your weight drops while you actually *enjoy* what you're eating. It really is possible to attain these goals without making your life more difficult or your diet more restrictive.

Finally, I would like to provide you with some insights into the bigger picture—how our food choices are affecting not only our own health, but also the health of the land, the environment, the animals, and ultimately our children. My goal is to help Americans create a healthier, more balanced relationship with food—and maybe at the same time to reallocate some of the money we are currently spending on weight loss to fund children's education and hunger projects, as well as environmental projects, and thus make a difference to the future of our planet. (I also hope to help some people who do not read this book: we will donate 5 percent of our profits to children's hunger programs and enivronmental projects.) Thank you for reading.

Part One

The Basic Principles

CHAPTER ONE

An Introduction to Ayurveda

Why Do You Crave What You Do?

*Positive health requires a knowledge of man's primary constitu-
tion and the powers of various foods, both those natural to them
and those resulting from human skill. But eating alone is not
enough for health. There must also be exercise, of which the
effects must likewise be known. The combination of these two
things makes regimen, when proper attention is given to the season of the year, the changes of the winds, the age of the individual and the situation of his home. If there is any deficiency of
food or exercise the body will fall sick.*

These are the words of the Greek physician Hippocrates, the father
of Western medicine, who lived in the fifth century B.C. and clearly
understood the connection of the body, the mind, and the environment, or the concept of healing the "whole person." As you will soon
understand, he might just as well be enunciating the principles of
Ayurveda. In his time it was called "humoral" medicine.

Ayurveda is an ancient, intuitive philosophy based on the observation of nature. Its concepts have been explained in full detail in many
books by many brilliant Ayurvedic physicians and practitioners. As a
nutritionist, I do not intend that to be the purpose of *Stop Your Crav-*

ings. I hope, of course, that you will become intrigued and want to learn more (if so, please see page 317). But the approach I take in my practice, and that I want to pass on to you, is not a completely traditional or classical approach to Ayurveda. For our purposes, you need to understand only four basic Ayurvedic principles that will allow you to use food as an ally in the ongoing battle against chronic dieting, obesity, poor health, and chronic frustration:

- The theory of the five elements.
- The theory of the three constitutional types.
- The theory of the six tastes.
- The theory of the six qualities of food.

I will explain how an understanding of these principles can help you to stop the cravings that have undermined your ability to stick to any diet plan you have tried.

The Balanced Approach was developed to help you create a simple and individualized plan based on food that tastes good and a lifestyle you can actually maintain over time because you want to, because it feels right, and because it gets you to your goals. *My* goal is to demystify the basic principles of Ayurveda and show you how they can be applied to an understanding of Western macronutrients—proteins, fats, and carbohydrates—food sensitivities, and overall digestive health.

To my knowledge, Ayurveda is unique in its ability to explain how to determine your own constitutional type and then use that knowledge in combination with an understanding of your physical and emotional imbalances to keep you, as an individual, in your particular life circumstances, as healthy, slim, and fit as you can possibly be. By knowing your constitutional type, you will gain insight into how you respond to stress, weather, even different times of day, and you will understand how all these factors affect your cravings and the foods you choose to eat. I have found that many people actually do know what they "should" be doing, but because they have been so bombarded with conflicting information, they become overwhelmed and no longer trust their own natural instincts or intelligence.

Like traditional Chinese medicine, Ayurveda looks upon digestion as the key to good health. In order to achieve optimum digestive health, it is first necessary to understand your own body so that you will be able to listen to the signals it is sending you and respond by providing it with the kind of fuel it needs to function at maximum efficiency. More often than not, when you experience an overwhelming craving for a particular kind of food—be it something sweet or something salty, or simply something warm and soothing—it's because your diet is lacking a nutrient that your body needs. In Ayurvedic terms, something in your system has gone out of balance. That imbalance may be caused by any number of factors: you may simply have been eating foods that were inappropriate for your constitutional type; you may have triggered a genetic food sensitivity by eating too much of one particular thing; you may have been affected by the weather or the changing seasons; or you may simply be under so much stress that you need to eat something that is soothing and nurturing.

Whatever the reason, if your diet is lacking a particular nutrient, chances are you will find yourself craving just that substance. Have you heard of pica syndrome? It describes people who compulsively eat nonfood substances such as dirt, clay, cornstarch, laundry detergent, or baking soda. Researchers have discovered that the syndrome occurs because these people's diets are deficient in the minerals contained in those substances, and they are subconsciously trying to obtain the nutrients they are missing. This is, of course, an extreme example, but here's another one that might hit closer to home. In an article "Chocolate: Food or Drug," published in the *Journal of the American Dietetic Association,* Kristen Bruinsma, M.S., and Douglas L. Taren, Ph.D., write, "Chocolate may be used by some as a form of self-medication for dietary deficiencies (e.g., magnesium) or to balance low levels of neurotransmitters involved in the regulation of mood, food intake, and compulsive behaviors (e.g., serotonin and dopamine)." Under normal circumstances, if you are anxious, your body will try to find a way to calm itself; if you are fatigued, it will find a way to be reenergized. In fact, that's usually what's happening when you reach for a Hershey's bar or a mocha latte at three or four o'clock in the afternoon.

So you see, our bodies are working all day long to keep us in balance. It's not just some odd, occult, or foreign notion. In Western terms, balance is referred to as "homeostasis," and the body's effort to maintain that condition is a constantly occurring natural process. It's actually what keeps us alive and our organs functioning. Seen from that point of view, hunger is simply a signal from your body that it needs more fuel. If we didn't experience hunger, we wouldn't know when to eat, and sooner or later we'd starve to death. If we didn't experience thirst, we wouldn't drink; eventually our kidneys would stop functioning, our electrolytes would be out of balance, and we'd wind up on dialysis.

According to the American Dietetic Association (ADA), a craving can be defined as "an intense, periodic motivation aimed at gaining the craved substance . . . this urgent inner demand overrides all others, undermines reason, resolve and will. . . . It does not stop until it is satisfied." The problem for many Americans is that we really don't know how to interpret the signals our body is sending us, or we have been taught to believe that ignoring our body's signals is a sign of strong character, even though, if you just look back at that definition of a craving, you'll see why this will never work. We believe that if we're hungry, we should just grit our teeth and tough it out; if we crave something sweet, it's a sign of weakness to give in. We've reached a point in this country where we've come to believe that everything is either "good" or "bad." Mainly, we're convinced the foods we crave are bad and those we force ourselves to eat are good. Coffee is bad, sugar is bad, salt is bad, fat is bad. No wonder more than 50 percent of us are overweight; we've simply been setting ourselves up for failure. It's only human nature to want what you can't have, and the more something is forbidden, the more desirable it becomes. What I hope *Stop Your Cravings* will help you to understand is that no food or nutrient is either good or bad unless you are consuming it in ways that are inappropriate. For example, coffee is not bad for you if you're in good health, you're not under stress, and you're sipping a cup after a meal or while relaxing at an outdoor café in Paris or Rome. But if you're exhausted, stressed beyond endurance, and gulping four cups to get yourself up in the morning or three cups to keep you going in the afternoon, you are not providing your body with the nutrients it needs, and the coffee, ultimately, will only make the situation worse.

Ayurveda provides the tools we need to learn how to listen attentively to the signals our body is sending us and how to respond by providing it with appropriate, nutritious fuel that will both satisfy our cravings (those all-important signals from our body) and keep our digestion running smoothly and efficiently so that we stay in balance (achieve optimum homeostasis).

Ayurveda is a theory based on thousands of years of observation. Its concepts may not be subject to proof by double-blind controlled studies, but once you understand them, you will know why you have been so frustrated for so long by unsuccessful diets and why you have been fighting your essential nature in order to "get thin."

THE THEORY OF THE FIVE ELEMENTS

The foundation of both Ayurveda and traditional Chinese medicine is the theory of the five elements. Basically, both philosophies maintain that we, and everything else in the universe, are made up of air, ether, fire, water, and earth. Everything from our body type to our personality type to the time of day, time of year, and time of life is connected to these five elements, and it is through these elements that we are connected to nature and the universe.

For the purposes of this book, the main thing you need to understand about the elements is that each has particular qualities. Think about the qualities of air: it is light, dry, and mobile. In Ayurveda they say that the air element is responsible for everything that moves in our bodies, from the blinking of our eyes to the movement of our muscles and joints. Ether, on the other hand, is defined as empty space. Think of a vase or a glass waiting to be filled with flowers or water. Air fills that space and makes it move.

Fire is obviously hot, and according to Ayurvedic principles, we would not be able to digest our food without the fire in our bellies, so fire is responsible for our metabolism. People who have a lot of fire in their makeup will share particular physical characteristics and personality traits, as do those with a predominance of air and ether.

Water is damp and mobile, while earth is grounded and heavy, and a combination of these two elements in the body will create an atmosphere that is thick, wet, and damp, just like congestion and excess fat.

Once you begin to understand how these elements combine to create your own constitutional individuality, you will come to see why your system operates the way it does, why you react to physical and mental stress in particular ways, and even why the changing seasons affect you as they do.

THE THREE CONSTITUTIONAL TYPES

To put it as simply as possible, the three basic constitutional types identified in Ayurveda are Vata (dominated by air and ether), Pitta (dominated by fire and water), and Kapha (dominated by earth and water). These "types" are determined by the particular physical and emotional characteristics or qualities that dominate each individual's body and mind. I have found that my clients gain tremendous insight into their own situation simply by understanding how the five elements relate to their own constitutional type. As I describe the attributes of each type, you will quickly come to understand why it is associated with these particular elements and, most important, why it is that the perfect fuel for one could be poison to another.

Vata (Air/Ether)

Vatas are the ectomorphs of the world. Physically, they tend to be thin, with delicate bone structure and low body fat. They usually have quick metabolisms, and they find it very difficult to put on size or build muscle. If Vatas have a weight problem, it's usually that they lose weight too quickly!

They are the people at the gyms who are frustrated because they don't generally have strong appetites and tend to stay skinny no matter how hard they train. Because Vata (air and ether) is responsible for movement, Vatas are drawn to aerobics, running, or spinning classes, but the problem is that they already move too much and don't need to lose weight. A combination of weight training and Yoga would be better for them, but they aren't attracted to these programs because they *just want to move* and literally can't sit still. Food in general is not very important to them. They don't have enough "fire" in their makeup to cause strong hunger signals and are likely to tell you that they simply "forgot to eat." If you need a visual image, think Calista Flockhart, Kate Moss, or David Hyde Pierce.

Because of the preponderance of air and ether elements, Vatas tend to have problems with cold and dryness. They suffer from problems like dry skin, dry hair, and brittle nails. They simply don't have enough body fat or lubrication to stay "well oiled" or warm.

When in balance, Vata personalities are quick thinking, fast talking, abstract, and creative—they might be artists, musicians, poets, or writers. They tend to be sensitive and spiritual, but because they have so much air and ether, they may also be a bit "spacey" and have trouble staying focused and grounded. They tend to be scattered and are often "running late." The routine of day to day is usually difficult for them.

In both Ayurveda and traditional Chinese medicine, the five elements correspond to specific organs and systems in the body. Vata is related to the nervous system, the bones, and the colon. Think about the qualities of each of these systems and organs and you will understand why. The term *nervous* is often associated with "flightiness"; the colon is associated with manufacturing air, gas, or "wind"; and the qualities of bone are dryness, porousness, and brittleness.

When Vatas are "out of balance," the imbalance is most likely to affect their nervous system. Under stress, they become anxious, worried, or fearful, and their feelings are easily hurt. They may be more sensitive, delicate, or spiritual than the other constitutional types. Physically, they are often subject to excess gas or constipation. As Vatas grow older, they are more likely than the larger, sturdier Kapha type to be prone to osteoporosis, again due to their slight, delicate bone structure and dry brittleness.

In Ayurveda, the time of year that correlates to Vata is fall into winter, when it is cold, dry, and windy, the leaves dry out, and then light, dry, fluffy snow begins to fall. The time of life associated with Vata is age sixty plus, when our skin and bodies become dry, brittle, and wrinkled. The Vata times of day are two to six A.M. and two to six P.M. Between two and six A.M. we are dreaming most actively, and according to Ayurveda, our brain should be most clear, abstract, and creative between two and six P.M. Because of the stress-filled American lifestyle, however, that is often the time when our blood sugar begins to drop, we aren't thinking clearly, and we desperately crave sweets and carbohydrates. When that happens, no matter what our "normal" constitutional type, we'd be experiencing a Vata imbalance. I'll be explaining how to handle that problem fairly easily.

Eating to Ground Your Vata

People who have too much air or gas in their system are considered to be in a Vata imbalance. This may be because they are naturally extreme Vatas or because external circumstances have put them in a Vata imbalance. If you are in a Vata imbalance, in addition to gas, bloating, and constipation, you may experience chills, shakiness, worry, nervousness, sleeplessness, difficulty concentrating, and inability to sit still or stop doing something. To be brought back into balance, your body needs to be warmed, calmed, lubricated, and nurtured. In other words, you need to eat foods that will counteract and "rebalance" your excess of Vata. To understand which foods will correct a Vata imbalance, you have only to think about the qualities or *energetics* of the food and what it is doing to your digestive system. (As a nutritionist, I was amazed by how much insight this philosophy provides into the qualities of food.) Beans, broccoli, cauliflower, lentils, popcorn, and rice cakes, for example, are all light, airy, and dry and therefore would tend to exacerbate rather than alleviate a Vata imbalance by adding even more gas or air to the system.

If you were suffering from gas or constipation, you wouldn't want to eat a meal comprising cold salad, raw vegetables, and beans. Yet many Vata constitutional types, possibly because they are often "sensitive" and spiritually oriented, tend to prefer vegetarianism, which means they may be choosing to eat exactly the foods that are wrong for them or preparing them incorrectly. While skinny Vatas can afford to eat more of the heavier carbohydrates, such as sweet potatoes, mashed potatoes, and grains, than other constitutional types, they also need plenty of good oils to lubricate them and balance their airy dryness. They need warm foods to counteract their tendency toward being cold, and they need heavier foods to calm them down and keep them grounded. Low-fat diets can be disastrous for Vatas, who actually need more good, monounsaturated oils and essential fatty acids than other body types, particularly if they live in a place where the climate is cold and dry. Remember that winter is the Vata time of year—the time when everyone needs to add more oils to their diet. And nature, in her wisdom, provides—nuts, winter squash, sweet potatoes, and other heavier, winter-type foods begin to appear in the markets just when our bodies need them.

This doesn't mean, however, that all Vatas belong on a meat-and-potatoes diet; on the contrary, a diet like that would probably be too heavy and put too much strain on their delicate digestive system. It does mean that Vatas, rather than eating their vegetables raw or cold, should sauté them in a bit of good oil, such as sesame or olive oil, or in butter or ghee ("clarified" butter from which the milk solids have been removed), and season them with carminative (gas-reducing) herbs and spices such as basil, oregano, ginger, cardamom, cinnamon, and cumin. They need foods that are warm, nurturing, nourishing, lubricating, and grounding, with sweet or salty and sour tastes. These might be warm, creamy soups; the lighter proteins such as eggs, fish, and cottage cheese; or mashed sweet potatoes with butter or ghee and nutmeg, cinnamon, or cardamom.

Pitta (Fire/Water)

We need fire to cook our food and, therefore, Pitta is said to be responsible not only for metabolism, but also for transformation and change.

Pittas are mesomorphs, with a medium frame and good genetics toward muscularity. They tend to get overheated easily and may retain water. For a visual image, picture Cindy Crawford, Tom Cruise, or Ted Turner. Pittas don't do well in warm, humid climates—take them to Colorado on vacation, but never to southern Florida, especially in the summer! They have strong appetites and good metabolisms; therefore, they get cranky if they miss a meal, and they *never* "forget" to eat. In fact, if they don't eat on schedule, they are likely to develop acid reflux or heartburn.

Pittas also tend to be type A personalities. When they are in balance, they are productive, organized, focused, "get it done" people with sharp minds and the capacity to work until they drop. Your Pitta friends are likely to be lawyers, stockbrokers, salespeople, or academics. They are absolutely *compelled* to "accomplish stuff."

When stress hits and Pittas are out of balance, however, they have a greater tendency than other types to become angry, frustrated, annoyed, irritable, and overly competitive. Physically, their imbalance usually affects the liver, gallbladder, spleen, blood, and eyes—the organs, according to traditional Chinese medicine and Ayurveda, that are related to heat. The liver, which is the organ most closely associated with Pitta, is the body's main detoxifying organ. When it is overloaded with toxins and can't process any more, the "poisons" may overflow into the bloodstream and come out through the skin, causing problems like acne, irritation, or redness. Everyone has heard alcohol referred to as "firewater," and most people know that too much alcohol over too many years leads to cirrhosis of the liver. It's the perfect metaphor for describing what can happen to the fiery Pitta. The conditions that Pittas develop are those related to heat: indigestion, heartburn, esophageal reflux, skin rashes or inflammations, canker sores, and hot flashes. When Pittas are out of balance, they just need to "calm and cool down" and cleanse and cool the liver.

The Pitta time of year is spring into summer, when the days are longest and the climate is hot and/or wet (think of spring floods and the dog days of August); the Pitta time of life is twenty to sixty years old, the time when we are most "fired up" and anxious to "make it"; and the Pitta times of day are ten A.M. to two P.M. (when the sun is highest and hottest) and ten P.M. to two A.M. During the first period, according to Ayurveda, the "digestive fire" is at its strongest, which is why, as I'll explain, you should be eating your largest meal in the middle of the day and a lighter meal in the evening (the Kapha time of day)—so that when your Pitta fire is again at its strongest, between ten P.M. and two A.M., your liver can perform its cleansing without also having to digest a heavy evening meal at the same time, which would undermine the efficiency of both functions. Have you ever stayed so late in your office that the cleaners couldn't get in to do their job? If so, you certainly noticed that when you arrived the next morning, the trash can was still overflowing and yesterday's garbage had not been removed. That's exactly what can happen to our bodies if we don't give our liver enough time to "empty the trash" during the night: it's still there when we get up the next morning, so that our stomach might be a bit bloated or our eyes red and puffy.

Eating to Cool Down Your Pitta

Pittas need to cool the fire in their belly. If you are naturally an extreme Pitta, or if you are currently in a Pitta imbalance—and it is important to remember that anyone, no matter what his or her natural type, can be put into a Pitta imbalance by external circumstances—you might experience diarrhea, skin rashes, burning eyes, increased appetite, overheating, and perspiration. You might find yourself engaging in compulsive, workaholic behavior, and you will probably feel frustrated and irritable. The foods that will correct a Pitta imbalance tend to be sweet and bitter as well as cold and astringent. Have you ever used aloe vera on a sunburn? It's cool and astringent and takes the fire out. Pittas, or those in a Pitta imbalance, do well with dark green leafy vegetables, such as kale, collard greens, and chard, all of which are bitter, as well as the more "cooling" proteins like cottage cheese and the lighter fishes. The fun part of combining Ayurveda with sports nutrition is that you will learn how to add spices, flavors, and simple chutneys to make your food taste irresistible, not bland and boring! Pittas tend to crave sweets and cold drinks as well as cool places. They may be the most uncomfortable and out of balance between the hours of ten and two, when the sun is at its highest and hottest; later in the day, they tend to relax and feel better again. To satisfy their craving for the sweet taste and its cooling effect, Pittas can enjoy flavoring their foods with sweeter herbs and spices like cardamom and fennel. On the other hand, they should avoid using excessive amounts of spices that are too heating—cloves, mustard, onion, chilies, radish, and cayenne. While too much red meat is excessively heating, other animal proteins, such as organic, free-range chicken and fish, may help to satisfy the Pitta's strong appetite and digestive fire. To counteract a Pitta imbalance, peppermint tea or a drink made up of cool spring water with cranberry juice and lime provides just the sweet and cooling combination to do the trick.

Kapha (Earth/Water)

If you mix earth and water, what do you get? Mud—a wonderful combination of elements that allows the flowers, food, and trees to grow, but one that is also heavy, damp, and thick.

Kaphas are endomorphs—larger body types who are not necessarily overweight, but who tend to gain weight more easily than they lose it, in part because they have a tendency to hold fat and water. In great shape and in balance, they might be large, strong football players and great athletes. For a visual, imagine Rosie O'Donnell, Oprah Winfrey, Drew Carey, or Dr. Andrew Weil. The Kapha appetite is steady but not as strong as that of Pitta types, and Kaphas may well miss a meal, but because they lack the Pitta's digestive fire, and because their metabolisms are most efficient at storing body fat, it is difficult for them to lose weight. In the hunter-gatherer days of our ancestors, they would have been the most efficiently designed for survival because their systems are made for storage. They are slower moving than the other types, with good endurance, and they prefer to avoid exercise of any kind.

Kapha is responsible for stability and solidity, and Kapha personalities tend to be strong, reliable, dependable, calm, and even-tempered; they may be the peacekeepers of the world. When all goes well, they are loving and compassionate, but when they are out of balance, they can be depressed and lethargic, sleeping too much and lacking in enthusiasm. They tend to hold on to both fat and emotions. These are the clients who come to me and lament, "I really don't overeat, I swear, but I just can't seem to get the weight off." This is an important point to understand. If you were born a Kapha, you are not going to look like a Vata no matter how much you diet or exercise. Ayurveda can help people understand and learn to accept their physical and emotional traits and then learn how to maximize their strengths and minimize their weaknesses. You don't want to have to "fight" with your body your whole life.

Physical problems in Kaphas tend to affect the chest and lungs. They can become congested and collect mucus, suffering from colds, asthma, bronchitis, or sinus infections.

The Kapha time of year is winter into spring, when it is cold and damp and when many people are suffering from colds, congestion, allergies, and sinus problems. Our bodies are actually designed to hold extra fat and mucus for insulation during the colder months, just as animals put on thicker coats. The Kapha time of life is zero to twenty years, when our bodies are anabolic—that is, growing and collecting tissue (remember all those runny noses and ear infections you had as a child?). By the time children reach the age of eighteen, they usually stop getting ear infections because they have "outgrown them" or, in Ayurvedic terms, have reached the Pitta stage of life, when their internal "fire" is burning off the excess mucus. But if you were to feed a stuffy-nosed child foods containing wheat, dairy, and gluten (the protein in oats, rye, barley, spelt, and kamut as well as in wheat), you'd only be exacerbating the problem. (Most adults know instinctively not to drink milk when they have a cold or are congested; wheat, gluten, and dairy can cause mucus or congestion in the body). The Kapha times of day are six to ten A.M. and six to ten P.M. Many of us, left to our own devices, would naturally go to sleep by nine or ten o'clock at night, and if you think about it, we are often a bit sluggish, perhaps a bit cold, even a bit congested, when we first get up. It takes us a while to be completely "up and running," which is also why, as we'll be discussing later on, early morning is the best time for some quiet meditation followed by exercise to "get the sleep out" so that we feel less sluggish and lethargic.

Eating to Fire Up the Kapha Metabolism

Kaphas need to be dried out and heated up. If you're in a Kapha imbalance, you might be feeling dull, heavy, and sluggish. You might be holding more weight than is comfortable or healthy for you. You'll be congested, and your symptoms will be at their worst in the morning and early evening. Some of the light and dry foods that will put a Kapha back in balance include quinoa, beans, and spinach. Beans and greens, in addition to being light and dry, are also astringent and therefore help to dry out the excess Kapha fluid. Cooking foods with heating, pungent spices and flavorings such as ginger, black pepper, mustard, cloves, cayenne, and jalapeños will also help set fire to the sluggish Kapha metabolism. It's interesting in this context to note where bodybuilding and Ayurveda come together: bodybuilders use thermogenic supplements, which contain heating herbs such as cayenne, ginger, and black pepper in addition to fat-mobilizing supplements to burn off body fat. Ayurveda would do the same thing by using specific exercises, foods, and herbs to "heat up" and "dry out" excess Kapha or congestion and body fat. The main difference in the Ayurvedic approach to weight loss is understanding your innate constitution in relation to your imbalance.

If heating, drying foods are helpful, those that are thick, wet, damp, sweet, and slow moving have the opposite effect. Dairy products like yogurt, cheese, and ice cream will only aggravate the Kapha tendency toward too much mucus and congestion, as will some gluten-based grains (especially wheat and oats) and hot cereals such as oatmeal. Many ethnic cuisines seem intuitively to add heating spices like lemongrass, basil, or red chilis to high-fat foods like coconut milk in order to "cut the fat" and aid digestion, and I've noticed that many people who are Kapha constitutional types seem to crave hot and spicy foods. That's just the body's natural intelligence at work.

Because Kaphas generally have more trouble than either of the other two constitutional types reducing body fat, they should follow a diet based mainly on light proteins such as fish and organic chicken, salads and lots of vegetables, nongluten grains, and beans cooked with small amounts of "good" (monounsaturated) oils such as sesame, walnut, or olive oil, and add additional essential fatty acids. They would do well to avoid the heavier, fattier proteins derived from red meat, as well as high-starch, glutinous, sticky carbohydrates like pastas and breads.

The chart below puts the differences among the types into graphic form so that you can see at a glance the determining characteristics just described.

THE BODY TYPES

	Vata	Pitta	Kapha
Element	Air, ether	Fire, water	Earth, water
Attributes	Cold, dry, mobile, moves a lot	Hot, wet, oily, medium tenacity	Thick, wet, damp, slow-moving, good endurance
Responsible for	Movement	Metabolism	Stability, solidity
Affects	Nervous system, bones, colon	Liver, gall bladder, spleen, small intestine, blood, eyes	Lungs, stomach, body fat, congestion, lymphatic system
Personality	Variable. Moves a lot. Always on the go, doesn't sit still for long. Attracted to aerobic exercise	Type A, strong personality. Talks fast and sharp	Calm, even-keeled. Not easily upset, worried, or irritated. Good at keeping peace
Body Type	Ectomorph. Poor muscle development, low body fat	Endomorph. Medium build. Good genetics for building muscle	Mesomorph. Holds body fat; hard to lose weight. Holds water
Appetite	Erratic. Often forgets to eat. Fast metabolism	Strong. Gets cranky if misses a meal. NEVER forgets to eat. Good metabolism	Slow. Slow metabolism. Can miss meals. May not overeat, but still holds body fat

THE BODY TYPES (continued)

	Vata	Pitta	Kapha
When Balanced	Creative, abstract, spiritual, sensitive, talks fast, moves quickly, fast mind, thinks a lot	Sharp mind, intelligent, single-focused, quick but sharper than Vata.	Strong, reliable, dependable, loving, calm, even keeled, good staying power
Qualities	Light, dry, cold, quick, variable	Hot; wet; feels warm; overheats easily; may hold heat and water in hot, humid climate	Cold, wet, damp, thick, mucousy, slow-moving
Physical Imbalance	Weight loss, too much movement, insomnia, dry skin, brittle nails, cold all the time, gas, bloating, constipation, can't wind down	Hot, irritable, high blood pressure, ulcers, ulcerative colitis, heart attacks, rashes, skin irritation, will work until ready to drop	Lethargic, overweight, congested, mucousy, sleeps too much, doesn't feel like exercising
Emotional Imbalance	Nervous, anxious, worried, fearful, sad, insecure, delicate, hypersensitive, overwhelmed	Angry, frustrated, annoyed, irritable, cranky, overly competitive, aggressive	Depressed, sad, feels sluggish, has no enthusiasm
Season	Fall–winter (cold, dry, windy)	Spring–summer (hot, wet)	Winter–spring (cold, wet, damp)
Time of Life	Age 60+ (dry, brittle, wrinkled)	20–60 years old (most fired up)	0–20 years old (growth and accumulation of tissue)
Time of Day	2–6 A.M., 2–6 P.M.	10 A.M.–2 P.M., 10 P.M.–2 A.M.	6–10 A.M., 6–10 P.M.
"Seat" of Body	Colon, bones	Small intestine, liver, spleen, gall bladder, blood, eyes	Lungs, stomach

In or Out of Balance

Now that you've had an overview of each of the three types, it's important for you to understand that each of us has all five elements within us. Most of us are a combination of types, perhaps one or two on a mental/emotional level and one or two on a physical level, so you might be a Pitta/Kapha body type and a Pitta/Vata personality type.

Some people are fairly equally balanced among the three, while others might be purely one, such as Vata, both physically and emotionally. It's also possible to be dominant in two types physically, two other types emotionally, and still have a third kind of imbalance. The self-test in the following chapter will allow you to determine your innate, genetically determined type or combination of types—that is, the type you are from birth (your legacy from your parents) and what you would be if you were in a perfect relationship, with the perfect job, in the perfect climate, and perfectly in balance both physically and emotionally. In Ayurveda, this is your *prakiti,* your birth constitution.

But most of us don't get to live in those perfect conditions very often, so it is essential that you pay attention not just to your innate birth type, but to the particular imbalance you are experiencing at any given moment. This is called your *vikriti.* You might, for example, be a Vata/Pitta body and personality type—with a small to medium build and a type A but slightly spacey personality, but if you were in a Kapha imbalance, you might have a cold or bronchitis or some other type of congestion. Or you might be a Vata/Pitta type who is also in a Vata imbalance, in which case you would probably be gassy or bloated and feeling scattered, overwhelmed, and "out of control." Because of the stress created by anything from our work to our family situation to the weather, the traffic, finances, or an infinite number of other external causes, most of us are almost always out of balance in one way or another. Even *good* stress, such as getting married or having a baby, can throw you out of balance. Of course, you need to determine your "birth" characteristics so that you don't inadvertently aggravate them, but you'll probably be spending most of your time learning how to detect balance and imbalance. The process of balancing is very important, but is dealt with incorrectly in Western medicine and sports nutrition. In Western nutrition, deprivation is applied to promote weight loss. Weight management is treated differently in Ayurveda. You need to determine whether you are a Kapha by birth, born to heavy parents, and heavy your whole life. Then you would treat the Kapha by trying to heat it up, stimulate it, and dry it out. But, if, on the other hand, you are a type A Pitta who has three kids, has been very stressed out and craving lots of sweets and cooling, calming foods, and who is now thirty pounds overweight, you are not a Kapha—you are a Pitta in a Kapha imbalance, and we would not want to overheat or overstimulate you any further.

We'd want to cool you down, calm and nurture you so that the cravings and body fat would eventually balance out on their own. Oprah could be an example here. She is a Kapha/Pitta with a pretty Vata lifestyle. She has mentioned on TV that when she gets upset or overwhelmed she craves lots of heavy comfort foods. In Ayurveda that is correct. She is not "bad" or lacking control, she's trying to calm and nurture herself. We'll be giving you advice on how to do that *without* undermining your digestion, gaining weight, and going on the binge, guilt, depression roller coaster. This example shows a key difference in the way Ayurveda deals with obesity and weight management. Understanding these differences has helped me to understand my clients much better and to help them take control of their weight and their health. It's about balance, not deprivation! One of the ways, according to Ayurveda, for the mind and body to bring themselves back into balance is through the six tastes and the six qualities of food. Food is considered therapeutic in Ayurveda and is therefore a significant component of any healing medical plan.

THE SIX TASTES AND SIX QUALITIES OF FOOD

The difference between the Balanced Approach program and other, more "conventional," approaches to weight management is the incorporation of the Ayurvedic theory of the six tastes and the six qualities of food.

Of course, you must still know how to balance proteins, fats, and carbohydrates in relation to your metabolic profile and activity level, and you need to understand the effects that food sensitivities, cultural diversity, and genetics can have on your overall health. But for me—and I hope for you—the "fun" part comes when you begin to understand how Ayurveda and most traditional ethnic cultures use herbs and spices to maximize digestion, enhance flavor, and balance emotions. And once you have learned that, you should no longer fall prey to the one universal pitfall encountered by virtually everyone trying to lose or control weight—*failure to comply with the program*. In the fitness world, I constantly hear complaints from trainers about how difficult it is to get their clients to stick to their high-protein, low-carbohydrate diets. But the fact is that people can eat just so much grilled chicken or canned tuna before they rebel and binge on chocolate, salty chips, or cookies because they are craving the sweet or salty taste. Craving sweet in Ayurveda is not a crime and should not translate into 80 pounds of white processed sugar or binging on tasteless "diet" cookies!

The Six Tastes

If you can remember as far back as your high school science class, you may recall that six distinct tastes—sweet, sour, salty, pungent, bitter, and astringent—can all be experienced on the tongue. From an Ayurvedic perspective, it is important to include all six of these tastes in every meal in proper amounts to stimulate, balance, and satisfy your particular constitutional type or imbalance. It's easy once you understand it. As I've already mentioned in the introduction to this book, most of the cuisines that we think of as "ethnic" or "European"—Chinese, Japanese, Mexican, Italian—do combine all these tastes in virtually every meal. A typical Asian meal would be a perfect example of this. It will normally include some protein, usually fish or tofu; some rice, which is *sweet;* ginger and wasabi, which are *pungent;* sautéed vegetables *(bitter)* cooked with sesame oil, a good, monounsaturated fat; soy sauce, which is *salty;* and green tea, a strong antioxidant that is both *bitter* and *astringent;* and a fruit, such as an orange (both *sweet* and *sour*), for dessert. Whenever I begin to describe to my clients the difference between this kind of typical Asian meal and the average American "diet" meal, I can see their eyes light up in anticipation. The Asian meal is clean, light, satisfying, healthy, and stimulating to the taste buds and digestion; turkey breast and a plain salad gets old really quickly.

The following chart lists the tastes of some common foods and how they affect the various constitutional types. In traditional Chinese medicine and Ayurveda all foods, herbs, and spices have a quality, a taste, and an effect on the body and the mind.

The Six Tastes and How They Affect the Body Types

Sweet: sugar; honey; milk; butter; cream; rice; breads; wheat; barley; ricotta cheese; tofu (soy); almonds; sesame seeds; meats; avocado; sweet fruits; the sweeter vegetables such as fennel, carrots, beets, winter squashes, yams, and cucumbers; spices such as fennel seed, cinnamon, cardamom, poppy seed, anise, dill, tarragon, fenugreek, and nutmeg

Sweet tastes are calming, moistening, and soothing. They are also anabolic, meaning that they help to add tissue, and, in excess, they will increase body weight.

Sour: yogurt and sour cream; lemons and other citrus fruits; fermented cheeses such as blue cheese; vinegar; pickles, tomatoes, plums, raspberries, strawberries, and unripe fruits

Sour tastes stimulate the appetite and digestion, increase metabolism, and help to dispel gas. They are also anabolic, meaning that they help to add tissue and, in excess, will increase body weight.

Salty: olives; soy sauce; tamari (soy sauce without wheat); kelp and other seaweeds; some salsas and fresh chutney; foods to which salt is added, such as chips or peanuts; sea salt, orsa salt, and celtic sea salt

Salty tastes are warming, calming, and drying. In small quantities they help to stimulate appetite and digestion, but too much can cause water retention; because they are also anabolic, they can increase tissue and body weight if eaten in excess. Celtic sea salt and orsa salt contain all the trace minerals from the ocean and do not promote water retention or raise blood pressure the way processed table salt can.

Pungent: wasabi (Japanese horseradish); chilies; peppers; garlic; mustard; radishes; onion; herbs and spices such as ginger, cayenne, cloves, rosemary, cinnamon, cardamom, cumin, coriander, thyme, sage, and turmeric

Pungent tastes are those we think of as spicy. They increase metabolism, circulation, and digestion and are also drying. Because they are catabolic, meaning that they help to burn fat, they can be helpful in lowering body fat, but too much can easily overheat a fiery Pitta.

Bitter: dark green leafy vegetables such as spinach, kale, collard greens, mustard greens; turmeric; eggplant; rhubarb; sesame; licorice; chocolate; beer; tonic water; coffee; tea; green tea

Bitter tastes are dry and cooling, small amounts help to stimulate digestion, and because they are catabolic, they can aid in reducing body fat.

Astringent: lentils; most beans; pomegranate; green apples; pears; cabbage; chard; spinach; rhubarb; green grapes; orange and lemon peels; herbs and spices such as thyme, nutmeg, sage, rosemary, cinnamon, coriander, caraway, bay leaf, basil, tarragon, and turmeric; aloe vera

Astringent tastes are drawing, drying, cooling, and catabolic, which means they aid in the reduction of body fat.

Each of the six tastes is also associated with the five elements:

Sweet = earth and water
Sour = earth and fire
Salty = water and fire
Pungent = fire and air
Bitter = air and ether
Astringent = air and earth

Because of these associations, each taste will also have a particular effect on each of the three body types:

To Decrease Vata: sweet, sour, salty
To Decrease Pitta: sweet, bitter, astringent
To Decrease Kapha: pungent, bitter, astringent

To Increase Vata: pungent, bitter, astringent
To Increase Pitta: pungent, sour, salty
To Increase Kapha: sweet, sour, salty

The above information is adapted from Ayurvedic Cooking for Westerners *by Amadea Morningstar, and* Ayurveda: The Science of Self-Healing *by Dr. Vasant Lad.*

Aside from their effect on each of the constitutional types, the primary reason the six tastes are so important is really quite simple: Variety and vivid flavors make eating more pleasurable. Many Americans seem to have forgotten this, or now believe anything that tastes good has to be "bad." Either we choose quantity over quality, or, at the other end of the spectrum, we restrict ourselves to bland, boring foods—such as a never-ending diet of grilled chicken and steamed broccoli—in the mistaken notion that this is the way to lose weight. But, in the end, neither of these ways of eating will accomplish the intended purpose, and that probably accounts, at least in part, for why so many Americans are overweight. I know, because I've been there myself. Every time I decided to "go on a diet," it was the same story: a quarter pound of turkey breast, one slice of whole-wheat bread, and a salad with no dressing. Invariably I'd be "good" from Monday to Friday and then "blow" it over the weekend. And I see the same pattern over and over again in my clients.

No matter how much you eat, if the food isn't full of flavor, and if it doesn't answer your natural cravings for all six tastes, your taste buds won't be satisfied and eventually you'll go looking for what you are missing—usually in the wrong places. A craving for salt will lead you directly to a bag of potato chips. Lusting for sweet? Your hand will go right for the cookie jar. That's why restrictive weight-loss diets never work and why, more often than not, even the most compulsive dieter will "pig out" by going on a binge and overeating. In Ayurveda, nonaddictive cravings are physiologically correct.

In fact, the best way to keep your weight under control and optimize your metabolism is to feed your body a *variety of nutritious, tasty fuel*. The key to utilizing nutrients efficiently and, at the same time, eliminating toxins is to keep the digestion strong. Taste, according to Ayurveda, is directly related to health, digestion, and satisfaction. The six tastes keep the digestive fire burning efficiently; bland, boring foods cause it to die down so that you are not metabolizing effectively. Just think about what happens when you have a cold—your nose is stuffy and you can't taste or smell. Therefore, you lose your appetite. In Ayurveda they would say that your digestive fire has "left its seat"; it is fighting a battle and therefore can't be used to process food at that time. As a result, your appetite decreases and your digestion becomes inefficient. But Ayurveda also believes the reverse is equally true: if your food is not full of vibrant and varied tastes, your appetite and digestion will eventually weaken because your taste buds are not being stimulated, toxins will accumulate in your digestive tract, you won't metabolize nutrients efficiently, and you may lose your health. Good taste, good digestion, and good health *always* go together in Ayurveda.

This doesn't mean, however, that we need to consume these tastes *in equal quantities* at every meal. Again, as with all aspects of Ayurveda, balance is key. As Amadea Morningstar points out in her book *Ayurvedic Cooking for Westerners,* "In Ayurveda it is often said, 'eat as much bitter and astringent taste as you like; have sweet and salty taste in smaller amounts; and sour and pungent foods in the least amounts.' . . . If you are craving astringent or bitter foods, you are likely to be needing them. Sweet and salty foods are easy to eat a bit too much of, and so Ayurveda reminds us to watch this. Sour and pungent foods include many which can inflame or irritate the gut; and so from an Ayurvedic view, the lesser, the better." But it all depends on your constitutional type and your imbalance. Vatas can have more heavy, oily, sweet, salty foods. We just want them to be of good quality.

So, always keeping an eye toward balance, using the full *variety* of tastes can add zest to your eating experience while *specific* tastes can help you to keep the digestive fire burning properly, which is one of the keys to achieving and maintaining ideal weight, increasing lean muscle, and decreasing body fat.

The best way to ensure that you are getting enough of the tastes that will balance your Vata, Pitta, and Kapha is to prepare your food with a variety of herbs and spices. Here's a list of a few that will probably be most familiar to all of you, along with their tastes and effects on the body. Chapter 10 will provide a wide variety of recipes for using them in exciting and flavorful ways. Remember, herbs and spices add taste, stimulate digestion, and can help mobilize body fat without adding additional calories or carbohydrates.

> *Basil:* Its taste is pungent and its effect on the body is heating. It will decrease Vata and Kapha, and in excess, it can increase Pitta.
>
> According to Ayurveda, basil can help to increase the clarity of the mind and open the heart, as well as boost the immune system. It can help to remove Kapha from the lungs and increase digestive fire. It is also helpful for removing Vata from the colon and can aid digestion.
>
> Fresh basil in pesto with olive oil, sea salt, and a small amount of garlic is excellent for all three constitutional types.

Black Pepper: Its taste is pungent and its effect is heating. It can decrease Vata and Kapha and, in excess, can increase and over-stimulate Pitta.

Black pepper is used as a digestive stimulant to burn up undigested food particles and cleanse the digestive tract of toxins.

Cardamom: Pungent and sweet, it has a heating effect. It decreases Vata and Kapha and, in excess, can increase Pitta.

Cardamom is one of the best digestive spices. It can aid in removing toxins from the system and in decreasing congestion and body fat, and it has been shown to help neutralize the negative effects of caffeine—which is why in India they put it in tea to make chai. In addition, it's very good for calming the nervous system and is especially wonderful in warm milk mixed with cinnamon and fennel or with cocoa. It's one of my favorites for calming cravings.

Cayenne: Its taste is pungent and its effect is heating. It decreases Vata and Kapha and increases Pitta.

Cayenne is a strong stimulant and good for heating up the digestive fire. It would be good for Kaphas who are trying to lose weight, as would other hot peppers. Too much cayenne can irritate the digestive tract, so you should pay attention to how you feel after eating it.

Chamomile: It is bitter and pungent and its effect is cooling.

Usually taken as a tea, chamomile is good for all constitutions but is especially cooling and soothing for Pittas. In addition to aiding digestion, it helps to clear the mind, balance the emotions, and calm the nervous system.

Cinnamon: It is pungent and astringent and sweet. Its effect is heating.

It decreases Vata and Kapha and, in excess, increases Pitta.

Cinnamon is excellent for increasing digestive fire and aiding circulation. Like ginger, it is considered a universal medicine in Ayurveda and is less irritating to Pitta than ginger might be. Used in combination with cardamom and cocoa and added to warm milk or almond milk, it can help to balance cravings for sweets and chocolate. And it helps to cut fat.

Coriander: Bitter and pungent, it has a cooling effect. Coriander helps to balance all three constitutional types.

It is especially good for digestion and, along with cumin and fennel, is particularly good for curing Pitta's digestive problems without being too heating. Coriander is a wonderful herb that can help to mobilize body fat and eliminate toxins while still being cooling to the digestive system; thus it can cut Kapha and cool Pitta at the same time, which means it is perfect for a type A personality who is also a bit overweight.

Cumin: Sweet, pungent, and astringent, cumin has a cooling effect and it helps to balance all three constitutional types.

Cumin dispels gas, aids digestion, and is restorative to the tissues. Like coriander, it decreases Kapha and also cools Pitta.

Try putting some in cottage cheese with a little cinnamon and a drop of maple syrup. Cumin, coriander, and fennel tea is a wonderful anti-Pitta, digestive drink (see page 263).

Fennel: It is sweet and pungent, with a cooling effect that balances all three constitutional types.

Fennel is one of the best herbs for balancing the digestive fire, which helps to mobilize body fat without heating up and aggravating Pitta. It also helps to dispel gas and calm Vata.

Many Indian restaurants keep a small bowl of fennel seeds near the door for people to use as an after-meal digestive aid, and Italians often serve braised or sautéed fennel as a vegetable side dish.

Garlic: Garlic is mainly pungent but actually contains all the tastes *except* sour. Its effect is heating, so it decreases Vata and Kapha and increases Pitta.

Garlic is considered rejuvenative in Ayurveda. It cleanses undigested food particles and other toxins from the system. It also helps to decrease congestions in the blood and lymphatic system, which is why it is considered to promote cardiovascular health. In excess, however, it can be aggravating, particularly to Pittas. (Clients have told me that it makes them feel "spacey" or gives them gas.) Garlic also can increase mental dullness in some people, but it can be grounding and calming for Vatas.

Ginger: Sweet and pungent, dry ginger has a heating effect that decreases Vata and Kapha and increases Pitta when used in excess. Fresh ginger, on the other hand, does not aggravate Pitta.

Like cinnamon, ginger is considered a universal medicine in Ayurveda. Taken with honey, it can decrease body fat and congestion. With rock candy or sugar, it can balance Pitta. With sea salt, it is excellent for Vatas.

Green tea with honey and fresh ginger is excellent for decreasing body fat, eliminating toxins, and increasing the digestive fire. Almost every ethnic culture uses ginger in their cooking. Crystallized ginger candy is one of my favorite treats. It's like a ginger gummy bear with a little sugar on the outside. It is good for digestion and satisfying after a meal with a little chai or tea. Very low in calories but rich in flavor, it helps to cut fat.

Mint: Mint is pungent and its effect is cooling. It decreases both Pitta and Kapha, and in excess, it can increase Vata.

Both peppermint and spearmint help to aid digestion and calm the nervous system.

Peppermint is a bit stronger than spearmint, and peppermint tea with honey and a piece of crystallized ginger can be a very satisfying way to end a meal. Eater's Digest tea (by Traditional Medicinal) is nice as well; it contains peppermint, spearmint, lemongrass, papaya, fennel, and other gentle digestive spices.

Nutmeg: Its taste is pungent and its effect is heating. It decreases Vata and Kapha and increases Pitta when used in excess.

Nutmeg helps digestion in the small intestine and is excellent for calming the nervous system. For Vatas, or anyone suffering from insomnia, warm milk with cinnamon, cardamom, ginger, and nutmeg can be an effective sleep aid.

Parsley: Pungent and bitter, it has a heating effect. It decreases Vata and Kapha and, in excess, increases Pitta.

In addition to being high in vitamins and minerals, parsley is a diuretic and can help with bloating and PMS.

Raspberries: Astringent and sweet, it has a cooling effect. Raspberry tea decreases Pitta and Kapha and can increase Vata in excess.

Raspberry has a positive effect on the colon and the female reproductive organs. It is cooling and soothing.

Sesame: Sesame is sweet and heating. It decreases Vata and, in excess, increases Pitta and Kapha.

Sesame oil is grounding and warming, and sesame seeds help to calm the mind and build and strengthen bones for Vatas.

Turmeric: Bitter, astringent, and pungent, turmeric is heating. It decreases Kapha and can increase Vata and Pitta when used to excess.

One of the most important herbs in Indian cooking, an excellent natural antibiotic and a strong antioxidant, turmeric is being studied at the Memorial Sloan-Kettering Cancer Center for its anticarcinogenic properties. It can increase digestion, improve the intestinal flora, purify the blood, cleanse the tissues, and aid in the digestion of proteins.

An excellent remedy for sore throats is to gargle with ¼ teaspoon turmeric, ¼ teaspoon sea salt, and 2 teaspoons lemon juice mixed into 3 ounces of warm water.

Following is a list of some additional herbs, spices, and flavorings you might enjoy or want to experiment with in your cooking.

Herb/Spice	Taste	Decreases	Increases
Allspice	pungent	Vata/Kapha	Pitta
Almond	sweet	Vata	Kapha/Pitta
Anise	pungent	Vata/Kapha	Pitta
Bay leaf	pungent	Vata/Kapha	Pitta
Caraway	pungent	Kapha/Vata	Pitta
Cloves	pungent	Vata/Kapha	Pitta
Coconut	sweet	Pitta/Vata	Kapha
Dill	bitter, pungent	Pitta/Kapha	Vata neutral
Honey	sweet, pungent, astringent	Vata/Kapha	Pitta
Lemon	sour	Vata/Pitta	Kapha neutral
Lemongrass	bitter, pungent	Pitta/Kapha	Vata neutral
Mace	sweet, pungent	Vata/Kapha	Pitta
Marjoram	pungent	Vata/Kapha	Pitta
Mustard seed	pungent	Vata/Kapha	Pitta
Onion	sweet, pungent	Vata/Kapha	Pitta
Oregano	pungent	Vata/Kapha	Pitta

Herb/Spice	Taste	Decreases	Increases
Paprika	pungent	Vata/Kapha	Pitta
Pomegranate	bitter, sweet, astringent	Pitta/Kapha	Vata neutral
Pumpkin seed	sweet	Vata	Pitta/Kapha
Rosemary	bitter, pungent	Vata/Kapha	Pitta
Saffron	bitter, sweet, pungent	Balances all three types	
Sage	bitter, pungent, astringent	Vata/Kapha	Pitta
Savory	pungent	Vata/Kapha	Pitta
Star anise	pungent	Vata/Kapha	Pitta
Tamarind	sour, sweet	Vata/Kapha	Pitta
Tarragon	bitter, pungent	Vata/Kapha	Pitta
Thyme	pungent	Vata/Kapha	Pitta
Watercress	pungent	Vata/Kapha	Pitta

The above information is taken from The Yoga of Herbs *by Dr. Vasant Lad.*

The Six Qualities

The theory of the six qualities of food complements and expands upon the theory of the six tastes. According to Ayurvedic philosophy, these qualities—heavy, light, oily, dry, hot, and cold—not only add their own variety to the foods you eat, they also, along with the six tastes, are instrumental in keeping your particular body type (Vata, Pitta, or Kapha) sailing on an even keel or returning it to peak efficiency if the balance should tip. Imagine you're feeling cold, sad, and overwhelmed. A cup of hot chocolate with cinnamon and cardamom might be just the sweet, warm, unctuous, soothing antidote you crave. But if you're constantly under that kind of stress, too many soothing hot chocolates could well undermine any weight management program you were following. A cup of warm vegetable soup, however, flavored with garam masala (a combination of cinnamon, cardamom, cloves, black pepper, and a number of other sweet, pungent flavors) and sea salt, will provide the same warm, grounding, sweet, and salty tastes and qualities and will stop your craving without adding too many calories.

The Six Qualities and How They Affect the Body Types

Heavy: cheese, yogurt; meat; wheat products; nuts; fish; eggs; honey; soybeans; beets, carrots, cucumbers; bananas, figs, melons, oranges, peaches, pears, plums; garlic, salt; brown rice, buckwheat, oats

Light: popcorn, rice and rice cakes, barley, corn, millet, rye; spinach, celery, lettuce, tomatoes, zucchini; chicken; apples

Oily: dairy products; fats, oils; almonds, cashews, peanuts, sunflower seeds; chicken, eggs; soybeans; coconut; garlic

Dry: barley, corn, millet, rye, rice cakes, buckwheat, popcorn; potatoes; beans; broccoli, celery, spinach; honey; pumpkin seeds

Hot: hot spices, chilies, jalapeños; hot drinks, alcohol, tobacco

Cold: cold drinks, cranberry juice with spring water and lime, ice cream, mint, sorbets

To Decrease Vata:	heavy, oily, hot
To Decrease Pitta:	cold, heavy, oily
To Decrease Kapha:	light, dry, hot
To Increase Vata:	light, dry, cold
To Increase Pitta:	hot, light, dry
To Increase Kapha:	heavy, oily, cold

The above information is adapted from Ayurvedic Cooking for Westerners *by Amadea Morningstar and* Ayurveda: The Science of Self-Healing *by Dr. Vasant Lad.*

MAINTAINING EMOTIONAL BALANCE WITH FOOD TASTES AND QUALITIES

It makes perfect sense, of course, that certain tastes and qualities of food either "increase" or "decrease" particular constitutional types. What we're all seeking is balance and stability. If our genetics and biochemistry are pushing us to one extreme or the other, we need to work against those tendencies to find the middle ground.

The human body is a wonderful, self-regulating machine, and despite the fact that virtually no one is innately a perfect combination of Vata, Pitta, and Kapha, under ideal circumstances we would all probably gravitate toward just the kinds of food we need to keep our body and mind in balance. Vatas would seek out heavier, oilier, sweet, or salty but nutritious foods. Pittas would gravitate toward sweet, cool foods to help control their fire. Kaphas would be eating dark green leafy vegetables and spicy curries. If we had a craving for ice cream, chocolate, or French fries, we'd eat a small portion and our craving would be satisfied.

But the truth is that most of us do not live in ideal circumstances. We live in a world full of stress and noise, with too much to do in too little time, in a climate that may not be ideal for our type. Consequently, most of us are *out of balance* much of the time. When my clients are craving sweets or chips, I tell them to ask themselves the following questions: Am I actually hungry, or am I bored or stressed out? Did I have a decent lunch, including something warm like soup, some good protein and fat, and vegetables with spices and flavor? Did I have something sweet to finish the meal, and did I leave the table feeling satisfied? This is how Europeans, in general, eat and probably why most European cultures have less incidence of obesity than we do in America. So if the answer to any of those questions is "No," you haven't been giving your body the fuel it needs and you've probably been consuming too many sweet or starchy carbohydrates, which means your blood sugar is swinging all over the place. It's time to eat something warm if this is the case, to soothe and satisfy you, sufficient protein to keep your blood sugar steady, and good fats and oils to keep you grounded, along with something sweet to calm you down. But if you did have a nice lunch with all the proper nutrients and you're still craving foods that are salty or sweet, you may be worried, stressed, overwhelmed, or angry about something. If you are in a Vata imbalance—stressed, fearful, or overwhelmed—you will probably find yourself craving sweet, sour, or salty foods or heavy, creamy, oily foods. Your desire for French fries, a mocha latte, or a candy bar would make perfect sense because your body would be trying to calm, nurture, and ground itself.

In fact, the external circumstances governing the lives of modern Americans have put most of us in an almost constant state of Vata or Pitta imbalance. And in our rush to soothe ourselves—to calm our

Vata or cool our Pitta—we too often eat "to bury unpleasant emotions," as Dr. Candace Pert, a research professor in the Department of Physiology and Biophysics at Georgetown University Medical Center in Washington, D.C., so clearly puts it in her book, *Molecules of Emotion.*

> By tuning into your emotions as information about your digestive process, you can develop your ability to know what your body needs in the way of nourishment and when. . . . Ask yourself: Do I feel hungry?—and wait for a feeling of hunger to occur before eating.
>
> . . . A craving for something sweet may be a signal that your brain needs fuel, so bite into a piece of fruit; a desire for a hamburger may be telling you that your body needs more protein, so add more animal and/or soy products to your diet.

I have found that many people seem to crave sweets and carbohydrates virtually all the time, simply because they are not eating enough protein and fat and are waiting too long between meals. Sometimes, when you're trying to be "good," less is not really better. By understanding the six tastes and six qualities of food and how they are related to the qualities of the five elements, you will be able to make an educated decision about which foods, herbs, and spices will bring you back into balance and nurture you without causing you to gain weight or ruining your digestion.

When You're Out of Balance

Picture this scenario: It's July in New York City, ninety-five degrees in the shade, and the humidity feels like more than 100 percent. It's three in the afternoon, there's a report you have to get out by five, and the air-conditioning in your office is on the fritz. The phone won't stop ringing, and your boss keeps sticking his head in your door asking when you're going to be finished.

In a situation like this, anyone, no matter what his or her innate constitutional type, would be in a Pitta imbalance. You'd be overheated, aggravated, frustrated, annoyed, and possibly longing for a mocha frappaccino, which is sweet (the milk and sugar), bitter and astringent (the coffee), cold (the ice), and heavy (the "frapp"). This particular set of circumstances would aggravate a Pitta type the most, but Vatas would be completely overwhelmed by it all and craving cookies or candy, and Kaphas would just hang in there and suffer, possibly gaining weight even if they didn't eat anything. But by remembering the particular tastes and qualities of food that would correct a Pitta imbalance, you could rebalance yourself emotionally and avoid dietary disaster. A cool peppermint tea, Vata or Pitta tea, a cranberry juice with club soda and lime, or a limeade (all calming, cool, sweet, and astringent) might just do the trick.

Or put yourself in one of these two situations:

You've been working on a project for more than a month and the deadline is fast approaching. You've been getting to the office by seven each morning and not leaving until after eight at night. You've flown cross-country twice in the last month. The phone is ringing with questions, the e-mails are pouring in, and you can't keep up with it all. By the time you get home at night you're so wound up you can't fall asleep, and now you're starting to have digestive problems as well. All in all, you're feeling overwhelmed, overtired, and constipated.

Or: You and your spouse/mate/partner have just split up, and you are overwhelmed with grief and anxiety. How are you going to pay the bills? What are you going to do with the house? How are the kids going to handle this? How are you ever going to meet someone new at this stage of life? What are the neighbors going to say, and what about your family? You feel alone and depressed, and there is no one around to offer support.

Either of these scenarios would put a tremendous strain on your nervous system—too many things going on, too much to worry about, not enough help and support—and in consequence you would be in a Vata imbalance. In fact, many of the clients who come into my practice are leading lives not unlike the ones just described. They are overworked, overwhelmed, and undernurtured. There's a reason they're craving food with sweet or salty tastes and heavy, oily qualities. They are trying to ground and nurture themselves. It's impossible to separate our emotions from the cravings they create, and, seen from the Ayurvedic point of view, those cravings are physiologically correct. What I want to do is show you how to use food and flavoring, herbs and spices, to help you manage stress rather than create further anxiety.

John Douillard, author of *The Three Season Diet,* has suggested that American fast food is actually the perfect antidote to our Vata/Pitta-imbalanced society. A burger and fries are oily, heavy, and salty; add the pickle, lettuce, cheese, onions, and "special sauce" and you have all six tastes, especially if you finish your meal with a sweet, creamy shake. Then you eat the whole thing in your car. A meal like that would offer the perfect "balance" for our stressed-out, fast-paced, Vata-imbalanced society, except for the fact that it offers virtually no nutrients and is totally devoid of life-supporting enzymes. Eating foods that are full of life force, energy, and nutrients is one of the most basic aspects of the Ayurvedic philosophy. As a substitute for that fast-food meal, for example, a cup of warm soup, a better-quality protein source with a few chips or cheese, a cup of chai tea, or a small piece of chocolate would provide the same tastes and qualities and would be nutritionally satisfying as well. The goal from an Ayurvedic perspective is to figure out what your cravings are trying to tell you, and find a satisfying, healthy way to calm and nurture them without being destructive to your weight and digestion. Cravings are not bad—food does not have to be boring!

THE ENERGY OF FOOD

According to Ayurveda, different kinds of food have different effects on our minds and bodies. The energy of the food will affect our energy as well. If you've seen the movies *Like Water for Chocolate, Woman on Top,* or *Chocolat,* you may already have begun to understand this concept.

Foods that are pure, clean, and fresh, such as organic fruits and vegetables, cheeses, and eggs, are called *sattvic,* or "pure," in Ayurveda and are said to increase our clarity, love, and awareness. They keep the mind running smoothly and efficiently.

Other foods, such as caffeine, hot spices, and red meats, are called *rajasic* and are said to stimulate and increase energy and movement. In excess, they can overstimulate the mind and adrenal glands and increase anger and frustration. If you're a sluggish Kapha, a little bit of this kind of stimulation might be just the ticket, but if you're already a type A Pitta personality or in a Pitta imbalance, or if you're a Vata who can't stop whirling and twirling, eating these kinds of foods will only aggravate the situation.

The third kind of energy or effect results from foods that slow you down, causing dullness and lethargy. These foods are called *tamasic* and include frozen, processed, and microwaved foods that are devoid of vitamins, minerals, and live enzymes; wine and alcohol fall into this category as well. For an overweight Kapha, these foods would certainly be counterproductive. For a type A Pitta or a Vata who needs to slow down, a glass of wine now and then might not be such a bad idea, but too much alcohol will aggravate the liver and increase Pitta, so once more, it's a question of balance.

The bottom line is that when we put foods of better quality, foods that are full of life, into our body, they will not only satisfy our taste buds and cravings but also help to optimize our mental and physical well-being.

BALANCING YOUR EMOTIONS AND YOUR PHYSICAL CONSTITUTION

As you now know, sweet, sour, salty, and heavy, oily, hot foods will calm a Vata imbalance. And sweet, bitter, astringent, and heavy, cool, oily foods will cool and calm a Pitta imbalance. But overconsumption of either of these combinations could eventually send anyone into a Kapha imbalance. What you need to do is learn if you're in a Vata/Pitta emotional imbalance and how to correct it without throwing yourself into a physical Kapha imbalance that would lead you to gain weight. That's where a balanced approach to food will help. Assuming you've been eating the proper foods at the proper intervals, so you know your imbalance is emotional and not physical, you might try a hot chocolate with ¼ teaspoon of cardamom and cinnamon; or drink warm soy, almond, skim, or whole milk, depending on your physical constitutional type; or a cup of chamomile tea with honey. Any of these combinations would offer the soothing combinations you crave without destroying your diet. There are also Vata, Pitta, and Kapha teas specifically formulated with the proper herbs for correcting particular imbalances. Again, that's the beauty of using culinary herbs and spices to provide nurturing and satisfaction, because—once again—they add no additional calories or carbohydrates.

The only other approach—the one that has been used all along by the American diet industry—is simply to keep saying no. But, as should now be abundantly clear to us all, that approach doesn't work. You can keep trying to treat the weight problem alone, but continued deprivation will only exacerbate the sadness or loneliness or depression that is all too often the underlying cause of overconsuming carbohydrates and sweets.

ACHIEVING A BALANCED AWARENESS

Armed with an understanding of four of the basic theories of Ayurveda and how they relate to one another, you will be able to sense when your body is going into an imbalance and what to eat in order to bring it back into balance more quickly without compromising nutrition. To quote from *Perfect Health* by Dr. Deepak Chopra, who has been instrumental in bringing an awareness of Ayurvedic theories to the mainstream Western population, "The guiding principle of Ayurveda is that the mind exerts the deepest influence on the body, and freedom from sickness depends upon contacting our own awareness, bringing it into balance, and then extending that balance to the body. This state of balanced awareness, more than any kind of physical immunity, creates a higher state of health."

To me, this is the one aspect of the balanced approach to nutrition, health, and fitness that has been missing from every other diet/nutrition program. Until you have gained insight into how your own system handles stress, cravings, and emotional imbalances, you will never get off the diet roller coaster. But once you have achieved this state of "balanced awareness," once you know how to use food and spices to balance your cravings, manage your stress, and satisfy your taste buds, you will be able to stay grounded instead of getting whipped around by outside forces. You will be like the proverbial kung fu master, understanding your own strengths and weaknesses, always seeking to stay centered no matter what is happening around you.

But first, you must determine (or confirm your suspicions about) which type or combination of types you are, physically and emotionally. You'll be able to do that by taking the *Stop Your Cravings* self-test in the following chapter.

CHAPTER TWO

Which Type Are You?

The *Stop Your Cravings* Self-Test

Getting information from your body—learning to understand what it needs—is the same as getting information from any other source. You must ask the right questions. By this time, you understand that your body type is more than just your shape; it actually determines your essential nature. It is built into your genes and acts as a blueprint for your physical, mental, and emotional functioning.

Now that you're familiar with how Ayurveda can provide the tools for you to understand why your body craves what it does, and how to stop those cravings by consuming good, nutritious, tasty fuel, you'll understand how important it is to determine whether you're a Vata, Pitta, or Kapha constitutional type or some combination of types, by taking the self-test that follows. Again, be aware that your innate constitution can be different from your imbalance. This is the first place people get confused reading about Ayurveda.

THE STOP YOUR CRAVINGS SELF-TEST

Most people are a combination of types and may be one physical and another emotional type. Please rate yourself in every category in each of the three columns, using the numerical scale:

1 = Not at all   2–4 = Sometimes, somewhat like me   5 = All the time, a lot like me

Vata	Pitta	Kapha

PHYSICAL CHARACTERISTICS

Physical Frame

Vata	Pitta	Kapha
__ 1. Small bones; delicate features; thin, do not gain weight easily; above or below average height.	__ 1. Moderate; well proportioned.	__ 1. Thick, large, solid frame; large boned.
__ 2. Prominent joints; find it difficult to develop muscle; irregular proportions.	__ 2. Good genetics for muscle definition; can add muscle fairly easily.	__ 2. Heavy, well-developed; rounded, stocky, gain weight easily.

Metabolism/Digestion

Vata	Pitta	Kapha
__ 3. Delicate digestion; may have tendency toward gas, bloating, or constipation.	__ 3. Digestion usually good; don't tolerate hot, spicy foods well; easily overheated or aggravated by certain foods, such as citrus, vinegar, and tomato sauce.	__ 3. Slow digestion; retain water; slow, sluggish metabolism.
__ 4. Fast metabolism; have difficulty keeping weight on, lose weight easily; digestion often poor.	__ 4. Medium to fast metabolism; become cranky or uncomfortable if don't eat when it is mealtime.	__ 4. Slow, efficient metabolism. Can skip meals without a lot of discomfort but still seem to retain weight and body fat.

Appetite

Vata	Pitta	Kapha
__ 5. Variable appetite; forget to eat; irregular eating habits; eat on the run.	__ 5. Strong appetite; can eat large quantities of food.	__ 5. Slow but steady; I eat slowly.
__ 6. May crave sweet, salty, sour, and mildly spicy foods or heavy, creamy, oily, foods such as chocolate or fast food; like warm, soupy, cooked foods and sauces.	__ 6. Crave sweet, cool foods and drinks; like bitter and sweet tastes, such as coffee with milk and sugar, ice cream, sweet fruits or sherbets, salads.	__ 6. Like warm, spicy foods, hot spices, vegetables, and beans.

THE STOP YOUR CRAVINGS SELF-TEST (continued)

Vata	Pitta	Kapha

Elimination

__ 7. Stool tends to be dry, hard; constipated.	__ 7. Regular; tendency toward loose bowels; soft, oily; one to three times per day.	__ 7. Thick, heavy, slow, but regular.

Strength/Energy/Physical Activity

__ 8. Like to move; always running around but tire easily; low stamina.	__ 8. Have medium strength; drawn toward moderate duration/intensity sports such as bodybuilding, weight training, mountain biking, sprinting, hiking.	__ 8. Strong, good stamina and endurance; good physical strength; steady energy.
__ 9. Very active; quick movements, but energy comes in bursts; need to rest, but find it difficult to wind down; hyperactive; can't sit still.	__ 9. Competitive by nature; aggressive; enjoy competitive sports or intense yoga practices.	__ 9. Don't like to exercise; would avoid it if possible; can be lethargic; less active but will follow regular exercise program once I start.

Sleep

__ 10. Irregular, interrupted; when out of balance, will have insomnia.	__ 10. Little but sound; six to seven hours are adequate and best.	__ 10. Deep and prolonged; must get at least eight to ten hours to be comfortable.
__ 11. Can't wind down; toss and turn; have difficulty falling asleep; prone to waking up between two and six A.M.	__ 11. Energy and clarity are highest in the morning; don't need a lot of sleep.	__ 11. Tend to oversleep; slow to get up; need time to have coffee and read the paper. Needs to go to bed early in order to awaken early.

Skin

__ 12. Tends to be rough, dry, cracking, wrinkled; may be more exacerbated in fall and winter; don't tolerate dry, cold weather.	__ 12. Soft, oily, red, sensitive; don't like hot, humid weather; perspires easily; tends to break out; rashes; acne, sunburns easily.	__ 12. Thick, moist, cool, whitish, smooth.

THE STOP YOUR CRAVINGS SELF-TEST (continued)

Vata	Pitta	Kapha
— 13. Tendency toward cold hands and feet.	__ 13. Tends to be hot; easily overheats.	__ 13. Cool, damp weather bothersome.

Hair

Vata	Pitta	Kapha
__ 14. Tends toward dry, curly, frizzy, thinning.	__ 14. Soft, oily; reddish, golden, yellow; straight; turns gray early; balding.	__ 14. Thick, abundant, luxurious, wavy.

Eyes

Vata	Pitta	Kapha
__ 15. Small, lashes fall out easily.	__ 15. Sharp, penetrating.	__ 15. Large, attractive; thick lashes.

Lips

Vata	Pitta	Kapha
__ 16. Prone to dryness; thin; crack easily.	__ 16. Soft, medium, rounded.	__ 16. Large, smooth, full.

Nails

Vata	Pitta	Kapha
__ 17. Brittle, thin, break easily.	__ 17. Medium strength; soft.	__ 17. Strong, thick.

Speech

Vata	Pitta	Kapha
__ 18. Fast, expressive; use a lot of hand gestures; talkative.	__ 18. Sharp, quick, to the point.	__ 18. Slow, methodical, melodic, less talkative or expressive.

MENTAL/EMOTIONAL CHARACTERISTICS

Vocation

Vata	Pitta	Kapha
__ 19. Musician, actor, writer, poet, artist, advertising, fashion. Athlete, healer, laborer, waitress.	__ 19. Salesperson, stockbroker, lawyer, athlete, entrepreneur, scientist, doctor, academic.	__ 19. Teacher, manager, judge, arbiter, entrepreneur, bookkeeper, diplomat, accountant, volunteer.

Emotional Temperament

Vata	Pitta	Kapha
__ 20. Usually enthusiastic, vivacious, and curious.	__ 20. Bright, intelligent, sharp minded.	__ 20. Sweet natured, serene, affectionate, calm, loving, compliant.

THE STOP YOUR CRAVINGS SELF-TEST (continued)

Vata	Pitta	Kapha
__ 21. When out of balance will be fearful, insecure, anxious, nervous, shaky, worried, overwhelmed, sad, heartbroken.	__ 21. When out of balance, can be aggressive, easily irritated; hot tempered but forget easily; can be critical in nature.	__ 22. When out of balance, too attached; don't let go easily; depressed, lethargic; in denial, stubborn.

Mind

Vata	Pitta	Kapha
__ 22. Creative, abstract, imaginative; psychically and spiritually sensitive; mind tends to be active, restless.	__ 22. Quick, sharp, intelligent; logical; opinionated, penetrating, argumentative.	__ 22. Calm, slow, placid disposition.
__ 23. Learn new things easily but forget easily. Better at theory than practical matters.	__ 23. Efficient, precise, accurate; friends think I am a perfectionist.	__ 23. Slower to learn than other people, but have excellent memory and good retention. Good with organization and details.
__ 24. Have difficulty making decisions; have a problem completing projects.	__ 24. Can be judgmental; easily aggravated or frustrated.	__ 24. Not easily ruffled, aggravated, or angered.

Dreams

Vata	Pitta	Kapha
__ 25. Fearful; dream of flying, movement.	__ 25. Fiery, angry, adventurous, violent, problem solving.	__ 25. Romantic, watery; dream of the ocean, rivers, swimming.

Imbalance Tendency

Vata	Pitta	Kapha
__ 26. Constipation, gas, bloating; take on too many projects; easily thrown off balance; nervousness, anxiety, insomnia, cracking joints; worried, sad, heartbroken, forlorn, overwhelmed.	__ 26. Inflammation, high blood pressure, hyper-tension, red rashes, hot flashes; skin irritation; anger, frustration, irritability; heart attack, ulcers.	__ 26. Congestion, water retention, excess mucus; depression, lethargy; weight gain, obesity; sleeping too much.
_____ Vata Total	_____ Pitta Total	_____ Kapha Total

EVALUATING YOUR ANSWERS

Add up your score in each of the three columns. The column in which you have the highest score will be your dominant type. The column in which you have the second-highest score will be your secondary type. If your scores relating to physical characteristics are higher in one column, and those relating to mental and emotional characteristics are higher in another, you may be a combination of one physical and a second emotional type.

It's important to remember, as we've already discussed, that no matter your type, you must pay attention to whatever imbalance you might be in at any given time and always "treat" the imbalance, keeping your genetic type in mind. If you are a Pitta with a Kapha imbalance, i.e., a fiery person who tends to get overheated but is now suffering from congestion, you might try some ginger tea with lemon and honey, but not so much that you become completely overheated. It's a dance between the elements, with balance in mind.

So now let's move on to learn how to combine these principles with Western nutrition.

CHAPTER THREE

The Balanced Approach to Clean Proteins, Good Fats, and Nongluten Carbohydrates

Your Metabolic Profile

Up to this point, you've discovered your own particular constitutional type, and you know how the six tastes and six qualities of food can help keep you, as an individual, more balanced and better able to handle stress. This means you have gained insight into one important component of your battle with food cravings—especially for sweets and other carbohydrates such as breads, cookies, and cakes. (I can't recall even one client who has ever called me to say he or she was having trouble with an intractable craving for broccoli or kale.)

You understand that to maintain good health and achieve ideal weight, you must look at the whole picture and take into account a variety of factors, including your diet, your work life, your personal relationships, your stress, and your level of activity, as well as the season and the time of day. All these variables can affect your ability to stay with your eating program or to "fall off" and begin to crave those salty chips and creamy mocha coffees. It might be useful to compare your ongoing effort to stay in balance with an airline pilot's maneuvering to stay on course: he is actually off course almost 90 percent of the time and is constantly making necessary adjustments, just as you must make adjustments to keep your body and emotions in balance.

Ayurveda includes all these variables, and it is the one major component of the Balanced Approach that I believe differentiates it from other health and fitness programs. There are, however, two more important variables that can affect your cravings. One of these is the contribution made by Western medical/sports nutrition to assessing the role played by proteins, fats, and carbohydrates in conquering cravings, reducing body fat, and regulating your "metabolic profile." The other is knowing how digestion, food sensitivities, cultural background, and blood type all relate to one another and how understanding them can help you manage your health and weight control. What I am going to do is help you to pull together all these variables and make them specific to your particular constitution and lifestyle so that you will realize when something is out of balance and thus be able to address the problem in a way that will keep you from falling off the tightrope.

AYURVEDA FOR MODERN TIMES

Ayurveda is a brilliant, intuitive, and ancient philosophy, but the fact is that we no longer inhabit the ancient world. Rather, we live in a diversified, modern, industrialized society with a different, more sedentary lifestyle; many more food choices, both good and bad; and a more sophisticated scientific knowledge of human biochemistry. Not only have we become more sedentary, but so have the animals from which we derive our proteins. When we were a hunter-gatherer culture, we might have had to chase down our food for days or work in the fields from sunrise to sunset, in addition to which, the animals we consumed for fat and protein were organic and totally range free, so that both animals and humans were quite naturally lean and chemical free. In his book *Native Nutrition,* Ronald Schmid, N.D., gives enlightening explanations of the ancestral diets eaten by many indigenous peoples, from Greenland Eskimos to North American Native Indians, to Australian Aborigines, to the Masai of Africa, to the Fiji islanders. In all cases, according to Dr. Schmid, these people ate more animal protein than we do—sometimes up to 75 percent of their total diet in the form of fish or wild game—along with greens, nuts, berries, and some fruits, depending on availability and season. The point is that none of these traditional people had access to the starchy carbohydrates, refined sugars, and processed foods we have today. Living in these societies and eating these kinds of foods made weight management rather simple. I see this even today every time I travel to Africa or South America. We, however, have complicated matters by living in a high-tech, high-stress, fast-paced society, with virtually unlimited access to chemically altered, over-processed, overrefined products that provide far less nutritional value.

In the past, farmers and others who lived off the land ate with the seasons and according to what they were able to hunt, catch, or trap. Their produce was not chemically "enhanced" or fertilized, and neither was the food that nourished their sources of animal protein. If there is one thing that virtually all the best-selling diet gurus agree upon, regardless of what regimen they recommend to "fix" the problem, it is that the primary cause of increased obesity and other diet-based diseases among Americans is our overconsumption of saturated fat, processed foods, refined sugar, and refined flour, or the so-called advanced cultural diet of our time. Dr. Schmid notes that the diseases affecting the "civilized white man"—dental diseases, obesity, heart disease, and cancer—are different from those affecting the indigenous peoples of Africa, whose meager diet of vegetables, beans, eggs, goat's and sometimes cow's milk may leave them subject to malaria or typhoid but who have virtually no heart disease or diabetes, not to mention obesity or osteoporosis.

We'll be discussing the impact of digestive differences and food sensitivities in the following two chapters; for now, let's concentrate on balancing ratios and types of proteins, fats, and carbohydrates. It remains fascinating to me how many people, despite the wealth of nutritional information available today, are still confused about which foods are protein and which carbohydrate and have very little understanding of the different kinds of fat. If you are in any doubt, see pages 66–70 for a quick and easy reference.

WHAT ARE CLEAN PROTEINS, GOOD FATS, AND NONGLUTEN CARBOHYDRATES?

You've probably noticed that the title of this chapter includes the terms *clean proteins, good fats,* and *nongluten carbohydrates.* Clean proteins are those derived from wild (not farm-raised) cold-water fish and seafood, from organic, range-fed animals that have not been filled with steroids and antibiotics, and from free-range eggs, organic cottage cheese, soy, and other beans that have been grown organically. In addition, it is not difficult to combine vegetarian sources of protein that do not contain gluten, dairy, or soy (all of which may be difficult for many Americans to digest) in order to create a complete protein source of all the essential amino acids. See page 67 for some suggested combinations. The more familiar I've become with the natural foods industry and the work being done by organizations like the Chefs Collaborative, the more I've come to realize how important it is for us to eat good-quality, clean food whenever possible.

Good fats are the monounsaturated fats and essential fatty acids that actually help you to mobilize body fat rather than store it. These fats can help to liquefy and remove the "bad" sticky fats that clog your arteries, and are they necessary for maintaining the health of your cells. We can obtain essential fatty acids directly from blue-green algae and seaweeds, from wild fish that have fed on sea plankton, and from meat or poultry that comes from animals raised on grass (their more natural diet) but not from those raised on grain. The February 2001 issue of *Today's Dietitian* reports that even the American Heart Association (AHA) has taken a new look at its dietary recommendations with regard to fat intake and concluded that "a diet high in unsaturated fat and low in saturated fat can be a viable alternative to a diet that is very low in total fat." The AHA also now recommends that "fish be consumed twice a week." The "quality" of fat is now being considered along with the quantity. Thirty percent total fat is still the recommendation, but the AHA is now discussing the incorporation of monounsaturated and essential fatty acids.

Nongluten carbohydrates are fruits and vegetables as well as those grains that do not contain the gluten protein found in wheat, wheat products, rye, barley, spelt, kamut, and oats. According to the Celiac Sprue Association, approximately one in every two thousand Americans has been diagnosed with a sensitivity to gluten, also known as celiac disease, and as many as one in every two hundred to four hundred may have difficulty digesting gluten. Gluten sensitivity can cause problems ranging from digestive disorders to allergies, asthma, arthritis, and weight problems.

Ayurveda is traditionally a vegetarian philosophy, and most East Indian people are genetically constituted to digest a diet that is higher in wheat as well as dairy. It is important to reiterate, however, that you must take into consideration your own heritage, metabolic profile, digestive ability, and activity level to determine what's best for you.

In chapter 5, we'll be discussing in detail the role that a sensitivity to gluten can play in digestive health and why it is best, in any case, to vary the sources of starchy carbohydrates. Meanwhile, suffice it to say that, as is always the case with issues pertaining to proper nutrition and digestion, determining the appropriate ratios of these nutrients is largely an individual matter. That said, there are some universal nutritional principles of which virtually all Americans need to be aware. Perhaps the first of these to have fallen by the wayside in recent years is an understanding of how we metabolize each of the three macronutrients and what biochemical effects they produce.

GOOD FATS/BAD FATS

In 1988, when the Surgeon General recommended that everyone strictly reduce their consumption of fat—particularly saturated fat— he didn't simply raise public consciousness, he set off an epidemic of fat phobia and, incidentally, created an economic boom for the manufacturers of fat-free, reduced-fat, and "lite" products of every variety. Penny Kris-Etherton, Ph.D., R.D., and a member of the dietary guideline committee for the AHA, states, "We thought we had all the answers when we were telling people to decrease fat . . . but that message simply did not work. People thought all they had to do was control fat in their diet and not worry about anything else. They thought that because something contained no fat, they could eat all they wanted. Even if it was high in calories, like marshmallows or soda."

As a result, one study conducted by the National Institutes of Health indicates that the number of Americans who are too obese, for example, to fit into an airline seat has risen 350 percent between the mid-1960s and the mid-1990s. In addition, *Scientific American* reports that we spend almost $46 billion annually on diseases related to overweight and obesity and that more than 20 percent of American children are now obese. Clearly, while low-fat diets have worked for some people with specific health conditions, they have failed the more than 50 percent of the population that is still overweight and, at the same time, quite possibly deficient, as we've mentioned, in "good" fats—the monounsaturated fats found in olive and canola oil, among others, and the essential fatty acids (EFAs) found mainly in cold-water fish, seaweed, and wild game (or, for vegetarians, in flaxseed, borage, black currant, or evening primrose oil)—that we need to avoid dry skin, hair, and nails, and also to mobilize body fat and help maintain cellular integrity.

Essential fatty acids, so critical for maintaining optimum health, *must,* in fact, be derived from dietary sources because our bodies do not manufacture them (that's the meaning of the term *essential*). The Eskimo population, for example, whose diet consists of up to 60 percent fat derived from cold-water fish and seal meat, has the lowest rate of heart disease in the world.

How can that be? In a way, the answer is quite simple. Despite the exhortations of low-fat advocates everywhere, simply eating fat will not make you fat. The reason for that, however, is not quite so simple. It relates to the way we metabolize, store, and burn protein, fats, and carbohydrates.

One of the main problems to occur when you are following a low-fat diet is that you will also be eating less protein, because protein almost always comes in combination with some kind of fat, and you will also be eating many more carbohydrates, simply in order to maintain your minimum daily caloric requirement. As a result, regardless of your constitution or metabolic profile, you may be subject to the blood sugar swings that result from the way your body metabolizes carbohydrates.

THE CARBOHYDRATE, GLUCOSE, BODY FAT CONNECTION

The first thing you must understand is that you metabolize all carbohydrates, regardless of their source, by turning them into glucose, which is sugar. The increased level of sugar in your blood will then signal your body to release insulin, which is the hormone responsible (among other functions) for removing glucose from the bloodstream to be stored as body fat or used for energy. Insulin, to put it succinctly, is the *storage* hormone.

Not only the amount but also the *kind* of carbohydrate you eat can affect both the quantity of insulin released and the speed with which it is released. The higher the carbohydrate is on the glycemic index, the greater the amount of insulin it will trigger and the faster that amount will be triggered. The glycemic index is the indicator of how quickly a carbohydrate is metabolized and enters the bloodstream. Generally speaking, the simpler or more refined carbohydrates are highest on the glycemic index. These consist mainly of breads, cakes, cookies, pastas, candy, and white sugar but also include some vegetables, such as beets and carrots, that are higher in sugar. Complex, or less refined, carbohydrates are derived mainly from fruits and vegetables, legumes, and beans. (See page 291 for a listing of foods and their place on the glycemic index.)

By consuming carbohydrates alone, you will elevate your blood glucose and your body will produce excess insulin, which will remove the glucose from your bloodstream to be either utilized as energy or stored as fat. Either way, your blood sugar level may drop dramatically within about an hour and a half of eating, and you may begin to feel shaky, light-headed, or sluggish.

If your first meal of the day consists of a large glass of fruit juice, cold cereal with skim milk, and a banana (the typical "healthy" American breakfast, comprising mainly carbohydrates), you will cause your blood sugar to spike as your body metabolizes the carbohydrates and turns them into glucose, then to drop as the insulin removes the glucose from your bloodstream. This happens because there is very little protein or fat in the meal, and a six-ounce glass of fresh-squeezed orange juice alone can contain up to six hundred calories. That's why so many people say that if they eat breakfast, they are "hungry all day" and why many of my clients tell me they feel better if they've had an omelet or a shake with some protein in it. By starting the day with so much sugar, you set yourself up for blood sugar swings all day long. If you were a Vata/Pitta endurance athlete who was going to burn off those carbohydrate calories, you wouldn't need to worry about gaining weight. But if you are sedentary, if you don't exercise, if you spend your day sitting at a desk or in front of a computer, your body will store the excess carbohydrates as fat and you will begin to gain weight—especially if you are a Kapha body type.

Even if you are burning off the glucose as energy rather than storing it as fat, you might still experience the drop in blood sugar that occurs when the glucose leaves your bloodstream. In addition to leaving you shaky and dizzy, this drop in blood sugar can cause excessive mood swings and cravings for additional carbohydrates—a consequence that can lead to what some people have come to call "carbohydrate addiction." In fact, what is actually happening is that, with the glucose no longer available in your bloodstream, your brain thinks it is going into starvation mode and begins to signal your body that there is an emergency. The only two nutrients that can cross the blood-brain barrier and provide fuel for the brain are glucose and glutamic acid. So when your brain is deprived of fuel, it will "panic," go into emergency mode, and demand sweets or carbohydrates *right now*. It's not truly an issue of being addicted to carbohydrates; rather, it's an issue of not providing your brain with the energy it needs to function. This is why you may have heard people say "I think I'm going brain dead" or "My brain is turning off" when they are hungry. Although said metaphorically, these statements are actually true, because when levels of blood sugar drop too low, the brain simply isn't working at its best. And when that happens, no matter how "good" you *intended* to be on your diet, your cravings will overcome your best intentions—because your brain needs more fuel.

So whatever your body type or level of activity, it would be better to have included some good fat and clean protein in that breakfast. If, instead of the high-carb breakfast of juice, cereal, skim milk, and banana (which, coincidentally, Ayurveda considers too much "Kapha" and a bad combination for digestion), you'd had a simple protein shake, or nongluten bread with almond butter, cinnamon, and a drop of maple syrup, or cheese and crackers, or cottage cheese with cinnamon, sunflower seeds, and strawberries, or—if you had more time—an omelet with some chopped sautéed vegetables such as spinach or onion or peppers, cooked in a bit of olive or canola oil, with some rice or almond or feta cheese, and maybe some salsa or chutney, you would be getting more protein, your blood sugar levels wouldn't spike, and you probably wouldn't be hungry or craving sugar again for about three hours, assuming you are not under severe stress or in a Vata or Pitta imbalance. And, as you can see, protein needn't always be derived from meat sources. Adequate protein can be derived from sources including eggs (one of the best sources of biologically available protein), cottage cheese, beans and cheese, or nuts and grains. Nuts, grains, and beans are certainly higher in starchy carbohydrates than eggs and cheese, so again, the appropriate choices for any individual will depend on his or her metabolism, constitution, activity level, and sport and weight-loss goals. For breakfast, however, any of the lighter, easy-to-digest, nonanimal protein sources would be appropriate. At lunch, when your digestion is strongest (the Pitta time of day), you should be eating your largest meal of the day, and that would be the time to include the heavier proteins as well. In chapter 7, we'll be providing some simple meal suggestions not only for breakfast, lunch, and dinner, but for between-meal snacks as well.

THE IMPORTANCE OF PROTEIN

If you put some protein—three to four ounces is usually sufficient— in your meal, your blood sugar will most likely remain steady for about three hours. Although protein does trigger the release of *some* insulin, it is much less than the amount triggered by carbohydrates. In addition, protein signals your body to produce an equal amount of the hormone glucagon, whose action is exactly opposite to that of insulin. Glucagon puts the body into nonstorage mode by signaling it to mobilize fat *into* the bloodstream, where it can be used as energy. By eating a small amount of protein, you will avoid the mood swings that result from depriving the brain of the energy it needs, and you should no longer crave the sweets that cause your blood sugar to spike and then fall—in addition to which you will significantly cut down on the amount of excess glucose available to be stored as body fat! You must remember that there's a difference between wanting a small amount of sweet taste at the end of a meal, which is natural and correct, and having a constant craving for candy, cookies, or chocolate due to low blood sugar, which is a problem that needs to be addressed by managing your protein, fat, and carbohydrate intake.

Once again, it's a matter of balance. Different foods have different effects on your body. Sugars and carbohydrates elevate insulin levels and promote the storage of glucose as fat in many individuals. Proteins cause much lower elevations of insulin and, at the same time, stimulate the production of glucagon, which mobilizes stored fat into the bloodstream to keep your blood sugar steady and to be used for energy. By consuming the proper ratios of proteins and carbohydrates, and the right types of carbohydrates for your specific needs, you maintain a balance between insulin and glucagon, maintain your blood sugar levels, and prevent the storage of excess fat. Remember our discussion of homeostasis back in chapter 1? That's precisely what your body is trying to achieve with this balancing act.

IN DEFENSE OF FAT

And if that's true, you're probably asking, what role does fat play in this biochemical dance? The answer is, exactly none. Fat is the only macronutrient that neither raises nor lowers levels of either insulin or glucagon. As an agent of either burning or storing energy, fat remains neutral. In fact, it is possible that by adding a small amount of fat to your carbohydrate intake, you might actually be lowering the resultant insulin spike. A person with adult-onset or diet-related (type II) diabetes, for example, would be better off eating a piece of cheese rather than a carrot. Even a small portion of full-fat ice cream might be a better choice than the same amount of a sorbet. Why? Because both the carrot and the sorbet are basically all sugar, with little or no protein or fat, so that an equal amount of either would actually contain more simple carbohydrate than would the cheese or ice cream. Take a look at the ice-cream containers in your local supermarket. Invariably, any reduced-fat ice cream will have more sugar added to make up for the fat that has been removed.

One of the biggest mistakes we seem to have made in America—and one of the main differences between our diet and that of most European countries—is that we have taken virtually *all* the fat out of too many foods and replaced it with additional sugar, carbohydrates, and artificial sweeteners. And many of us have been storing all that excess sugar as fat. People were made to think they could eat as many of these low-fat foods as they wanted. Everyone began overconsuming "diet" cookies and other reduced-fat products, and we actually became even fatter.

So all fat is not, after all, the evil demon we've been made to think it is. Even saturated fat, which has been implicated as the villain in our ongoing battle with cholesterol, may not be so bad after all. In fact, cholesterol is not even a fat; it's actually a sterol or alcohol, a waxy substance that is necessary for many metabolic functions. And most of the cholesterol in our system is manufactured by our own cells; only about 30 percent or less comes from our diet. When the body manufactures too much, that, of course, can create a problem as the cholesterol begins to clog the arteries, leading to increased risk of blood clots, stroke, or a heart attack. And that problem would certainly be exacerbated by consuming too much saturated fat, which is gooey or, in Ayurvedic terms, excessively Kapha. So please don't misunderstand me: If you have clogged arteries, you certainly need to be careful of how much saturated fat you consume. And you certainly don't want to block a clogged artery even further by eating a big glob of cheese or lots of pizza.

But what triggers our body to manufacture excess cholesterol? Once again, it is related to elevated insulin levels. So too much insulin in the bloodstream (caused by too much carbohydrate in the diet) can, in certain individuals—particularly those with a family history of heart disease, diabetes, elevated blood pressure, and obesity—trigger the production of excessive amounts of cholesterol and triglycerides.

But cholesterol levels that are too low can also be a problem. We all need a certain amount of cholesterol, because without it we cannot produce adequate amounts of the two most important sex hormones, estrogen and testosterone. In addition, cholesterol provides the structural framework for all our cells; it helps to move nutrients into the cells and waste products out, as well as to move fats in and out of the circulatory system. Adequate cholesterol is also necessary to digest fats, because it is one of the main components of the bile acids that are secreted by the pancreas and the liver; and without it we would not be able to absorb the fat-soluble vitamins A, D, E, and K. So again, as with everything we've discussed thus far, it's a matter of achieving the proper balance. For that reason, I always suggest that my clients have a blood panel done before they start my (or any new dietary) program and then get retested in three to six months to be sure they're moving in the right direction.

While cholesterol levels should be neither too high nor too low, the more important issue to consider is the ratio of "good" (HDL) to "bad" (LDL) cholesterol. LDL is actually the lipoprotein that promotes cholesterol storage, while HDL is the component that helps to remove it. So in addition to a good overall cholesterol level, what you want to achieve is a good ratio of HDL to LDL cholesterol. And although it's still hard for many people to believe, it's actually *good fat* that can help you to achieve this.

The "Good" Guys

Aside from saturated (animal) fat, there are the monounsaturated fats and essential fatty acids we've already mentioned, one of whose necessary biological functions is to help "liquefy" the plaque deposited in the arteries by dietary saturated fats and the cholesterol manufactured by the body. Simply put, there are essentially two kinds of fat—those that remain solid at body temperature and those that remain liquid (this is the difference between fats and oils, the difference between lard and olive oil). Those that remain sticky and solid (or Kapha) are the ones that promote excess production of the "bad" cholesterol and triglycerides that clog up your arteries and lead to heart disease.

Even skinny, athletic people can have genetically high overall cholesterol levels because their bodies manufacture too much of it, regardless of the amount of saturated fat in their diet, and the only way to mobilize that fat out of the body without taking medication is to "melt" it. Fats do not dissolve in water, they clump up—remember what we say about two people who absolutely rub each other the wrong way? They're like "oil and water." Fat does, however, dissolve in fat. If you put a pat of butter in a pot of water, it won't melt without heat; but if you put a pat of butter in some olive oil, it will emulsify, or "break up." So adding those monounsaturated fats and essential fatty acids to our diet (the ones that remain liquid at body temperature) actually encourages the liquefaction of sticky plaque so that it can be "unstuck" from the arterial walls and then, with the addition of adequate fiber, be eliminated. (We need the fiber to move the fat along after it's been liquefied, and the fiber of choice for many Americans has, for a long time, been oat bran. But oat bran contains gluten, which can, in excess, cause digestive problems in some people. There are, however, Ayurvedic herbs, which we'll discuss in chapter 11, that will do the job without the gluten.)

Finally, fat is also necessary for maintaining the health of all the cells in our body. The main components of our cellular walls, along with cholesterol, are phospholipids, a kind of fatty acid. Lecithin, for example, is a phospholipid derived from soy that helps both to lower body fat and to increase cellular integrity. Phospholipids form the barrier that keeps things belonging inside the cell inside and prevents the entry of substances that do not belong inside (such as toxins). Obviously, without sufficient phospholipids, we cannot maintain cellular integrity. The weaker the cell walls, the more likely it is that toxins will penetrate, and the less able we will be to fight off disease.

Many studies have shown a correlation between a deficiency of good fats and problems ranging from attention deficit disorder (ADD) to premenstrual syndrome (PMS) to arthritis to prostate cancer and exacerbated menopausal symptoms, to mention a few (because these good fats are anti-inflammatory and help to lubricate the system). The solution, once again, is to determine what is causing the problem to begin with. A qualified nutritionist or herbalist might well be able to help you lower body fat, triglycerides, and cholesterol without depriving you of the good fats your body really needs.

For those of you who would like a more in-depth explanation of all the roles fats play in body chemistry, I suggest Udo Erasmus's brilliant book, *Fats That Heal, Fats That Kill,* which may give you more information than you ever wanted or needed to know about fat, but which is also easy and fascinating to read.

BALANCE IS KEY

So if protein keeps blood sugar levels even, and fat helps to maintain cellular integrity as well as to liquefy and mobilize plaque and reduce inflammation, why are we eating carbohydrates at all? In fact, there are some, most prominently Dr. Robert Atkins, who say we'd do better without them. Dr. Atkins's diet, which eliminates carbohydrate intake almost entirely while increasing levels of protein and fat, encourages higher levels of glucagon production, which puts the body into fat-burning mode while drastically reducing the amount of insulin available to encourage fat storage. As a result, many people have seen dramatically reduced levels of cholesterol, triglycerides, and body fat in a short time, which can be very exciting and motivating, especially for impatient Pitta-type Americans.

But this, like the very low-fat diet, is also extremely restrictive, and many people find it difficult to adhere to over a long period of time.

As John Douillard so astutely points out in *The Three-Season Diet,* whenever you remove any whole food group from your diet for an extended period of time, your body will eventually start to crave what is missing—even if it's fruits and vegetables over steak and fries. What we're trying to do here is provide you with a lifetime program that will not completely deny you *anything* and will help to acknowledge and balance your cravings, not increase them. In addition, there are some health concerns about the long-term effects of eating these extremely high quantities of fat and protein, especially if their sources are not organic (even Dr. Atkins now advocates eating organic). Many of these foods also contain large quantities of antibiotics and hormones.

One of the reasons this kind of diet produces such quick results in so many people is that it encourages quick and increased loss of water weight. Each gram of stored carbohydrate is capable of holding three grams of water; so when we eliminate all stored carbohydrates, the water has nothing to cling to and must be eliminated from the system. As a result, we begin to urinate with extreme frequency. In addition, the end product of protein metabolism is nitrogen and uric acid, which must be eliminated through the urine. The combination of eliminating carbohydrates and increasing proteins will result in frequent urination and thus a rapid initial loss of water weight. So even if we lost four to six pounds in one week, two of those pounds might be actual body fat and the rest would most likely be water weight.

Physiologically, it's almost impossible to lose more than two to three pounds of actual body fat in one week's time because, as I'm sure most dieters know, to gain or lose a pound of body fat we must increase or decrease our diet by a total of 3,500 calories (which equals one pound of body fat), and it is simply not possible to reduce your caloric intake by more than 7,000 to 10,000 calories a week. (You *should not* have to be counting calories in any case. It is not necessary and creates needless anxiety and neurosis.) When I get clients to move their bigger meal to lunch, eat every three hours, and have a light dinner, calories take care of themselves.

Any diet that reduces the caloric intake enough to induce a weight loss greater than 2 to 3 pounds a week is most likely so restrictive that it will actually cause your metabolism to slow down (because your body will think it is starving), which will eventually cause the diet to stop working. Ultimately you will gain back the weight you lost, as do

90 percent of all dieters, and you will once more be on the yo-yo diet merry-go-round, which will actually make you fatter over time.

In addition to the water loss, after about three to four days on a diet that is completely devoid of carbohydrates, the body will have depleted its carbohydrate stores, go into a metabolic shift—a condition called "ketosis"—and begin burning fat instead of carbohydrate for energy. Ketones are chemicals created as a byproduct of the liver's metabolism of fats. Normally the body is very efficient about removing ketones from the bloodstream, but when we eliminate all carbohydrates from our diet and must burn fat instead for energy, the ketones build up faster than the body can completely eliminate them, leading to ketosis. Some people, such as Dr. Peter D'Adamo, who advocates different diets for people with different blood types, theorize that certain populations—such as Native Americans or others with type O blood who were traditionally hunter-gatherers—might actually do well in a slightly ketotic state; but there is also evidence to show that a prolonged state of ketosis can lead to certain health problems, because while most of our systems can use ketones as fuel, the brain, red blood cells, and muscles used for rapid movement do not utilize them very well.

I do know many type O bodybuilders who seem to thrive on a diet that is high in protein and who say that they would never make it as vegetarians (who knows, maybe they were hunter-gatherer warriors in their past lives), and many bodybuilding experts do recommend this kind of high-protein, high-fat diet for a limited time—usually twenty-one to twenty-five days—to jump-start their clients' programs. I do believe, however, that even serious bodybuilders would benefit from a modified Mediterranean diet. On this kind of diet, you'd still be eating plenty of proteins and good fats, but you would also be incorporating a lot of the vegetables that are lower on the glycemic index, and you'd be flavoring your food with plenty of herbs and spices to satisfy your taste. You really can satisfy your cravings—as I'll be saying over and over again—without adding any calories or starchy carbohydrates to your diet!

And, once again, satisfying those cravings is key. Aside from the risks posed by ketosis, a diet completely lacking in carbohydrates, in my experience, can sometimes lead to depression, which is caused by reduced levels of serotonin in the brain. It is carbohydrates, as we have already discussed, that provide the glucose needed to raise serotonin levels, and, deprived of this particular nutrient, our bodies sooner or later will be crying out for—craving—something sweet or something high in carbohydrates. This is why, after two or three weeks, even highly motivated weight-training and bodybuilding clients (I see this more in women, most likely because of fluctuating hormonal levels) cheat on this diet or go on a binge to prevent their serotonin levels from dropping too low.

Most recently, Barry Sears, Ph.D., author of *The Zone,* has sought to balance the extremes by advocating a diet based on approximately 40 percent of calories from complex carbohydrates, 30 percent from protein, and 30 percent from fat, with some variations in these recommendations depending on your level of activity.

Dr. Sears does an outstanding job of explaining the health benefits gained by obtaining adequate protein and good fats, but what his book doesn't take into consideration are the differences in constitutional, biological, and metabolic types or digestive factors that are addressed by Ayurveda. Many books do talk about blood sugar swings, but they don't seem to know how to help people manage food under stress or to understand what it means to be in a Vata or Pitta imbalance. They can't seem to help people conquer their cravings and satisfy their desire for sweets by maintaining adequate serotonin levels while still encouraging the metabolism of body fat and aiding digestion. All of this is made possible by understanding the "qualities" or "energies" of different foods as well as how to use herbs and spices.

If all it took were the understanding that too much processed sugar was bad for us, the problem would have been solved by now. As a nutritionist, however, I have seen hundreds of clients who have read every diet book on the market and who are still confused and unable to balance their cravings, especially when they are under stress. Speaking with these clients, I am constantly reminded of Ayurveda's unique ability to interface with modern science and provide answers that are available nowhere else.

WHERE DO YOU HOLD YOUR FAT?
UNDERSTANDING YOUR METABOLIC PROFILE

There's no doubt that it's important for each person to obtain the proper balance of nutrients from proteins, fats, and carbohydrates.

But that balance will vary, depending on each individual's constitutional type as well as his or her lifestyle and level of activity. For example, a thin, active Vata or someone in a Vata imbalance would not only be able to metabolize more carbohydrates, but would also need more fat (especially in the winter months) than a fiery Pitta, whose liver might be overtaxed by metabolizing too much fat. Fortunately, there is an enormous amount of information, both in Ayurveda and in the scientific literature, relating to the ways people of different body types metabolize nutrients.

In terms of body type, medical science has shown that one important variable is the actual shape of your body or, to put it another way, where you tend to hold your fat. The population can be divided into two basic body shapes: "apples," or those who hold their fat mainly in the face and upper body; and "pears," those who have slim shoulders, waist, and abdomens but hold their fat mainly in the hips and derriere.

If You're an Apple

Too much fat stored in the upper body can be dangerous, because the fat also invades essential organs—primarily the heart. And it has also been proven that there is a strong correlation between people who store fat mainly in the upper body and those who are insulin resistant. Being insulin resistant means that you require more insulin than usual to remove excess glucose from the bloodstream because your pancreas may have become overworked and exhausted from trying to metabolize too many starchy, refined carbohydrates and too much sugar for too long. Storing upper-body fat has been correlated with specific diseases associated with insulin resistance, including heart disease; high blood pressure; type II diabetes; elevated levels of cholesterol, triglycerides, or other fats in the blood; and/or a tendency to retain fluids. People who store fat this way need to be particularly careful of the type and amount of carbohydrate they consume. I know this firsthand, because I am one of those who stores fat primarily in my face and abdomen.

People who are insulin resistant usually do better on a diet that is significantly lower in the starchy carbohydrates, such as breads, cakes, and pasta, and higher in lean, clean proteins and good fats.

This is basically the diet that follows the Mediterranean food pyramid: fish, occasional lean organic meats, olive oil and essential fatty acids, lots of vegetables and salads, and occasional small amounts of nongluten grain (depending on your activity level), all flavored with good, fresh herbs and spices. This type of diet will usually keep an insulin-resistant, apple-shaped Pitta or Kapha constitutional type in balance, lean and mean, with good digestion and good energy.

Following this diet, you might be consuming 20 percent to 30 percent of your calories from fat, but it will be "good" monounsaturated fat and essential fatty acids. And the fresh, preferably organic meats and vegetables, herbs, and spices you are eating will taste better and be more satisfying so that you will require less at every meal.

Personally, if I stick to this diet, my cholesterol remains midline or average and my weight—or percentage of body fat—remains lower. If I eat too many starchy carbs, both start to go up. I know when I have to cut back, but it's also possible to go too far in the other direction and consume too many essential fatty acids, in which case both cholesterol and body fat might actually start to drop too low. This is actually the goal of many elite athletes. It's a question of arriving at the correct balance of insulin and glucagon, as we discussed earlier. Once you understand this, you too will be able to tell when you can handle more carbs and when you need to cut back. You will be in charge of your body rather than out of control. Ultimately it's a question of tailoring your diet not only to your body type, but also to your goals and activity level.

But what if you're insulin resistant and store fat easily but are also a Pitta/Kapha who needs a certain amount of sweet taste to remain calm, cool, and collected? Once again, that's where Ayurveda can help by adding sweet flavors like cinnamon and cardamom, mango chutney, garam masala, or peanut satay sauce, among others, to your food, or drinking peppermint tea with honey. Eating a small amount of a healthy sweet such as crystallized ginger or good chocolate or a couple of yogurt-covered almonds—should calm your cravings for sweets without causing you to compromise your diet by consuming excessive amounts of starchy carbohydrates, like cookies, refined white sugar, and calories. And as we've said before, these flavors and spices will help your digestion to become more efficient, which will ultimately enable you to burn more body fat. In Appendix A I'll also be giving you recommendations for some organic candies that will help keep your sweet tooth happy with truly minimal amounts of carbohydrates.

What About Pears?

While people who store fat more equally above and below the waist, or predominantly in the hips and derriere, don't have to be quite so diligent about watching their carbohydrate intake, pear-shaped people need to pay more attention to specific training, supplements, and techniques that stimulate lower body fat. Having said that, it is true that virtually anyone would actually do well on a Mediterranean type of diet. It is a diet that traditionally changes seasonally as different products become naturally available, which is exactly what Ayurveda and traditional Chinese medicine advocate. It depends on the honest, clean flavors of nutrient-rich foods, and it is endlessly adjustable. Pittas would add more cooling fruits in the summer, for example, and all of us, but especially Vatas, would eat heavier proteins, along with more fats and oils, in the fall and winter. Even many modern chefs—and I'll be giving you some of their recipes in chapter 10— are now dedicated to preparing meals with ingredients that are actually in season, locally grown, and raised organically. It's helpful to us for maintaining balance and definitely better for the environment not to be shipping out-of-season products across the globe.

THE WISDOM OF EATING WITH THE SEASONS

You'll actually notice, once you start to pay attention, that your metabolism changes with the seasons. One summer, for example, when I was trying to be "good," keeping my carbohydrates low and my good fat and protein intake higher, I found myself, on a hot July day, cranky and clearly in a Pitta imbalance. The thought of tuna fish for lunch and pumpkin seeds (which I normally love) for a snack became totally unacceptable. All I could think about was watermelon. I resisted for two days, not wanting to break my low-carbohydrate diet, until finally, of course, my body overruled me and I had two big, sweet, juicy pieces of watermelon. I felt better immediately—happy, cool, and collected—and I didn't gain two hundred pounds or an additional 20 percent body fat. I had just needed to cool down—it was *July*, after all—and my brain had been trying to contradict the natural intelligence of my body. In the winter, I don't need or crave watermelon, and you probably don't, either.

Winter is the time when we look for warm soups, and I'll be explaining how to flavor them with heating, "thermogenic" spices like ginger, cloves, and cardamom that will help to minimize the excess body fat we naturally tend to collect during the colder months. It's also when nuts and seeds and sweet potatoes and squashes show up in the market, when squirrels start storing up nuts and animals put on heavier coats. We humans, too, might put on a pound or two to help us keep warm—and in most cases that's okay, because the weight should fall off naturally when we go back to eating lighter foods the next spring. It's all part of the natural cycle.

Vegetarian vs. Nonvegetarian

While I believe it would be nice if everyone on earth were vegetarian, I also know that isn't going to happen any time soon. That is why this book is combining Ayurveda with information on metabolic types and cultural differences. Different diets work for different people. We need to take diversification into account when we discuss health, weight loss, and nutrition. For many constitutional types, vegetarianism might not even be the healthiest kind of diet. (I've tried it more than once and have always, eventually, had to put some fish back in my diet. I can't metabolize all those carbohydrates.) It is possible to keep your protein intake high without eating meat. I would, however, urge you, whenever possible, to buy fresh, seasonal foods produced by people who are trying to create more compassionate environments for animals and to farm organically. Not only will the foods they produce be more flavorful and nutritious, which will be good for you, but you will also be doing something good for the animals and the environment. We will talk more about these issues in the final chapter.

SUMMING UP: THE MEETING OF EAST AND WEST

Looking back to the Ayurvedic theory of constitutional types, we see how the ancient wisdom of the East once more ties in to the modern science of the West. Vata types don't have much body fat to begin with, and they also burn fat quickly, whereas Pittas can hold a bit more fat but also tend to be more muscular, and Kaphas tend to both accumulate and store body fat very efficiently. In modern terms, we need to understand that different metabolisms utilize macronutrients differently.

In his book, *Ayurvedic Zone Diet,* Dr. Dennis Thompson overlays an understanding of Vata, Pitta, and Kapha onto the work done by Barry Sears in *The Zone* to arrive at ratios of proteins, fats, and carbohydrates that can be helpful to each constitutional type. In chapter 7, I'll be giving you plenty of suggestions for tasty and satisfying meals that help you to balance those nutrients.

The Vata Zone

As we've said, Vatas, because their constitution is genetically light, dry, and airy, and because they have fast metabolisms, need more oil to stay well lubricated and sufficient protein to ground them and keep their blood sugar stable. In addition, they are quite efficient at burning carbohydrates and can benefit from the grounding qualities of sweet potatoes, yams, squash, and even French fries. As a result, according to Dr. Thompson, this type might do best on a diet that is approximately 20 percent protein; 40 percent to 50 percent carbohydrate, depending on activity level; and 30 percent to 40 percent fat, derived primarily from ghee (clarified butter) and olive, walnut, or sesame oil.

The Pitta Zone

Those who are, in Ayurvedic terms, extreme high Pittas, on the other hand, may do better on a diet that is closer to 30 percent protein; 40 percent to 50 percent carbohydrate made up mainly of cooling salads, bitter greens with spices and sweet chutneys, and very small amounts of nongluten grains; and 20 percent to 30 percent cooling fats such as olive oil, along with essential fatty acids, because they are the people most likely to have a problem digesting fat. Remember that the organs related to Pitta are the liver and the gallbladder and that these are also the organs responsible for metabolizing fat. To stay cool and keep their digestive fire from burning too hot, they do better on the lighter proteins such as fish, eggs (egg whites are cooling and the yolks are heating, but using them whole is more balanced), cottage cheese (which is cooling), and lean, organic meats. And, as always, activity level and lifestyle come into play. Even the American Dietetic Association now agrees that weight-training athletes, for example, may need to eat more protein because they become more metabolically active. And even though I personally have difficulty metabolizing starchy carbohydrates, if I hike eight to ten hours, or if I snowshoe, cross-country ski, or whitewater kayak for four to five hours, I can eat as many carbs as I like. For me, French fries or good-quality potato chips that are salty but don't contain hydrogenated fats and are also wheat and gluten free would be my carbs of choice.

The Kapha Zone

Kaphas, according to Dr. Thompson, are the ones who do best on the 40 percent carbohydrate, 30 percent protein, 30 percent fat diet. Their fats should be monounsaturated olive and sesame oils, along with essential fatty acids to help them break down and mobilize stored body fat (remember what we've discussed about good fats helping to mobilize fat). They don't need a lot of protein derived from the heavier meats or from dairy products that would increase their tendency toward heaviness and congestion, but should get their protein mainly from fish, organic chicken and turkey, grains like quinoa and buckwheat, and beans. They should also eat lots of salads and sautéed green vegetables. And, of course, they should flavor their food with good, heating, pungent spices such as ginger, wasabi, and cayenne to dry them out and fire up their digestion.

How Much Is Enough?

Having discussed ratios of proteins, fats, and carbohydrates, I've found, in working with my clients, how difficult it is for many people to actually determine the *amounts* of various macronutrients they are eating. While the Balanced Approach to eating is not about weighing your food or obsessively counting calories—and eating a larger lunch and a smaller dinner, as I've already mentioned, should alleviate your worries altogether—I've found that the following equivalency charts can be helpful in giving people some parameters. In addition, you can consult the lists in chapter 1 to determine what effect these foods will have on your constitutional type or on any imbalance you might be experiencing.

Protein

Try to use wild fish and organic, free-range, hormone- and antibiotic-free meats and dairy products whenever possible.

Three to 4 ounces of protein is a portion about the size of your fist. I've found that eating this amount every 3 to 4 hours, with a larger, 4- to 6-ounce portion at lunch, should keep your blood sugar steady throughout the day and maximize digestion, energy, and weight management.

One ounce of protein contains approximately 7 grams. Exchanges for variety are:

1 ounce fish, chicken, turkey, beef, or pork
2 ounces firm tofu
3 ounces soft tofu
2 ounces cooked, or ¾ ounce dry uncooked beans, peas, or lentils
1 whole egg
3 egg whites
¼ cup egg substitute
¼ cup regular cottage cheese
⅓ cup low-fat cottage cheese
½ cup nonfat cottage cheese
¾ ounce hard cheese
1 slice packaged, presliced cheese
2 slices low-fat or nonfat packaged, presliced cheese

Complementary Vegetarian Protein Sources

Complete proteins are those that contain all of the essential amino acids and are derived from a single source, either animal or soy based. *It is easy to create complete proteins by combining nonwheat sources that won't aggravate your digestion or your Kapha. Here are a few nonwheat, nongluten, nonsoy, non–cow's milk alternatives.*

Grains and Nuts or Seeds

Rice and sesame seeds
Rice or millet bread and nut butter, such as almond, peanut, or cashew, or tahini
Rice protein and almond milk
Quinoa macaroni and almond cheese
Nongluten bread and almond cheese

Seeds and Legumes (beans, peas, or lentils)

Sesame seeds and garbanzo beans (chickpeas)
Pea soup and garbanzo beans or lentils

Grains and Legumes (beans, peas, or lentils)

Lentils and rice, quinoa, millet, amaranth, or buckwheat
Black or pinto beans and rice, quinoa, millet, amaranth, or buckwheat
Beans and corn tortillas (add feta, rice, or almond cheese for additional protein)
Pea soup and rice cheese (it's gooey and good for Vatas and Pittas)

Carbohydrates (Fruits, Vegetables, and Grains)

All fruits and vegetables are carbohydrate—the issue is really one of high glycemic index versus low glycemic index. It isn't necessary to measure quantities of most fruits and vegetables, but try to eat more that are lower on the glycemic index, such as dark greens, and less of those at the top, such as corn, beets, carrots, and sweet fruits. Or, if you do eat the sweeter carbohydrates, be sure they are cooked in good fat, with spices added for digestion, and eat them in combination with some protein. Vatas can include more of the heavy carbs than either Pittas or Kaphas. For a listing of these sources of carbohydrate, see page 291.

One serving of carbohydrates is approximately 20 grams, which means:

2 cups salad greens
2 cups dark green leafy vegetables and most green vegetables
1 cup frozen mixed vegetables (peas, corn, carrots)
1 cup berries
½ piece of fruit (pear, peach, apple, etc.)
2 cups *edamame* soybeans
1 slice packaged, presliced bread or ½ small bagel
1 (1-ounce) roll
½ English muffin
6 saltine crackers
3 graham crackers
6 Health Valley rice bran crackers (wheat and gluten free, one of
   my favorites)
3 cups air-cooked popcorn
2 rice cakes
1 or 2 ounces potato chips (nonhydrogenated)
½ cup corn kernels
1 small corn on the cob
⅓ ounce cold cereal (try nongluten)
½ cup cooked hot cereal (try nongluten, such as quinoa, buckwheat, amaranth, or millet)
3 ounces cooked sweet potato
4 ounces cooked white potato
1 cup winter squash
2 ounces cooked beans, lentils, or peas
½ cup cooked grain

It is better for many people to choose a grain that does not contain gluten. And while there are certainly those for whom gluten intolerance is not a problem, I would always suggest rotating your sources of grains and starchy carbohydrates to optimize digestion and nutrient intake.

Nongluten grains include rice, millet, quinoa (one of the best grains), amaranth, buckwheat, and corn.

Gluten grains include wheat, oats, rye, barley, spelt, and kamut.

Fats

One serving of fat is approximately 15 grams, which means 1 table-spoon, no matter what the variety of pure fat:

Essential Fatty Acids (must be acquired from dietary sources): omega-3s and omega-6s

EPA/DHA: from cold-water fish such as salmon, trout, mackerel, sardines, and fish oil capsules (eat wild fish 2 to 3 times a week)

Alpha-linolenic acid: flaxseed oil, hemp seed, and walnut oil (1 to 3 teaspoons or 2 to 6 capsules daily)

DHA: from blue-green algae, spirulina (can be taken in supplement form), and fish oils (such as salmon and sardine oils)

Linolenic acid: from flax, sunflower, safflower, corn, hemp, soybean, and walnut oils (use sparingly)

GLA: from evening primrose and borage oil, black currant, and pumpkin seed oil

Total EFAs: a blend of flax, evening primrose oil, borage oil, and lecithin (can be taken in supplement form)

Sources of Monounsaturated Fats

Olive oil
Avocado
Almonds
Sesame seeds
Peanuts
Olives

Sources of Saturated Fats

Whole dairy products
Butter or ghee
Mayonnaise
Meats
Poultry
Eggs

It's best to obtain most of your fat from monounsaturated sources and essential fatty acids and to limit your intake of saturated fats.

Avoid

Hydrogenated fats, found in baked goods and other products to increase their shelf life, can increase your risk of arteriosclerosis, which is associated with heart disease. Trans-fatty acids, found in margarines, have been shown to have carcinogenic effects.

By shopping in health food stores or buying from the companies listed on page 299, you can find chips, crackers, and cookies that do not contain hydrogenated fats and/or trans-fatty acids.

THE BOTTOM LINE

The goal is to achieve the proper balance of macronutrients for your own lifestyle and constitutional type—choosing the right ratios of clean proteins, good fats, and nongluten, nonstarchy carbohydrates to keep your body and mind functioning at optimum levels of efficiency.

For the average person (serious athletes obviously need more), no matter what his or her constitutional type, this would mean a lunch consisting of approximately four to six ounces of some kind of protein with some good fat added and about three ounces more protein every three hours to mobilize body fat, keep blood sugar levels in balance, and avoid those cravings for brain-calming sweets. The amount and type of carbohydrate will depend on your lifestyle and constitutional type, but in every instance, those carbohydrates that are lowest on the glycemic index will be the ones least likely to spike blood sugar levels and cause sweet cravings.

When it comes to carbohydrate intake, perhaps the best thing you can do for your health is to eat plenty of green vegetables. Not only are they low in calories and low on the glycemic index, they are also full of vitamins, minerals, antioxidants, and fiber. There is also ample evidence to show that eating plentiful quantities of cruciferous vegetables such as broccoli and cauliflower can help guard against diseases like cancer and heart disease. And always remember, whatever your ratios of macronutrients, to make your meals nurturing and satisfying by flavoring them with plenty of tasty herbs and spices. One of the reasons many people don't eat their greens is that they think they taste bitter (they are bitter—that's why they help with weight management and digestion) and may be difficult to digest for Vatas. Just adding a little good fat, wonderful spices, and a bit of sweet chutney will get you to think about vegetables in a whole new way. My clients are now cooking and truly enjoying kale, chard, collards, bok choy, mustard greens, and other leafy greens they never would have considered before learning to prepare them "the Ayurvedic way." By eating this way, you too will be able to balance your Vata, Pitta, or Kapha while making your taste buds dance.

As always in Ayurveda, the first premise is to eat what you can digest, which is what we'll be discussing in the following chapter.

CHAPTER FOUR

Digestion Is Key

Maximizing Health, Wellness, and Weight Management Through Optimal Digestion

By now we've already talked a lot about digestion and about the ways that balancing your diet with a variety of tastes and qualities of food, as well as the proper ratios of clean proteins, good fats, and nonstarchy carbohydrates, can ensure maximum digestive efficiency, thereby helping to promote optimal weight and maximum health. In this chapter and the one that follows, we'll be discussing how digestion actually works and how even "healthy" and nutritious foods may lead to digestive difficulties if they are not the appropriate foods for your individual biological type.

As Sarasvati Buhrman, Ph.D., co-founder of the Rocky Mountain Institute for Yoga and Ayurveda, explains, Ayurveda looks upon digestion as "the very root of health." Most Westerners, however, including most Western physicians, fail to consider digestion when assessing a health problem or complaint. Perhaps as a result of this, we in America are facing what could conceivably be considered an epidemic of digestive disorders. Sales of antacids like Tums and Rolaids are skyrocketing, indigestion is a household word, and there are statistics to indicate that a large percentage of the American population suffers from some type of chronic digestive disorder. The key issue in Ayurveda—and it should be the key issue for all of us—is not whether the food you eat is "good" or "bad," but whether or not you can digest it. In other words, you are what you absorb, not necessarily what you eat. If you are unable to process it, it isn't good for *you.*

Do you occasionally or chronically feel heavy, bloated, and have gas? Vatas, as we've said, are most likely to experience gas, bloating, constipation, and dryness in the colon because of the excess air and ether elements in their system. Or do you suffer from indigestion, gastric reflux, acid stomach, or ulcerative colitis, the complaints most likely to affect the fiery Pitta metabolism? In either case, it simply isn't "normal" to live with these symptoms, even though many Americans think it is. I have seen clients who have actually been constipated since childhood or who consider taking a Tums the appropriate conclusion to every meal.

Think of your digestive system as the engine of your car. If the engine isn't running properly, the car will be sluggish, the engine won't "purr." The same is true of your gut. If you're filling it up with the wrong fuel for its particular model or make, it will have to work harder to keep on running, and you won't be cruising at optimum speed. In fact, most people seem to be more in tune with the "health" of their car's engine than they are with their own digestive health.

In Ayurveda there are two important principles relating to digestion. The first of these is *agni,* which translates literally to mean "digestive fire" (or "metabolic fire"). *Agni* is responsible for helping you digest your food. Vatas and Kaphas find that they must work to maintain sufficient fire, whereas Pitta people may sometimes experience excessive appetite or excess fire, leading them to eat more than they can actually digest. If you were camping and wanted to put out a fire, you could use either earth or water, the two elements associated with Kapha. So Kaphas, even though they may not eat much, have too little fire to burn up the fat and wind up storing everything as excess. That's why some people say "All I have to do is look at food and I gain weight." Many Kaphas really don't overeat; they just store what they do eat really well. Vatas, on the other hand, because they have too much air and too little fire, don't feel hungry and may "space out" on eating because they get caught up in some other activity, and then crave sweets and suffer from blood sugar swings. Pitta, like *agni,* is associated with fire, and when Pittas are in balance their fire burns efficiently and their appetites are strong. When they are out of balance, however, their fire may be too hot, and that can also lead to problems. The goal is to "balance *agni*," to keep the fire burning without either letting it get too hot or allowing it to die down too far.

When your digestive fire isn't hot enough, or if it is so hot that you eat more than you can digest, you may begin to experience *ama*. *Ama* is the second important principle of Ayurveda related to digestion. It is the uncooked or undigested food particles that cause toxic buildup in your system. Ayurveda teaches that *ama*, or undigested toxic material, is one of the primary causes of disease. Have you ever noticed that when you are sick or have a cold, your tongue develops a whitish coating? That's a sign that your digestive tract is coated with mucus, which acts as a magnet for sticky, undigested food particles that slow down your digestion. But *ama* can also be caused, in a Pitta person, by an excess of bile (a yellowish or greenish liquid secreted by the liver that aids in digestion). Whatever its cause, it will make you sick and disrupt your digestion. Most animals and children won't eat when they're sick. In fact, if you live with a pet, you'll know that refusing food is one of your first clues that something is wrong.

Losing one's appetite or refusing to eat is the body's instinctive reaction to illness. When your system is infected with any kind of hostile agent, such as a virus or bacteria, most of your "fire," or energy, must be devoted to fighting the enemy, so there will be little fire left to devote to digestion. This is one reason why physicians trained in complementary/integrative medicine don't recommend aspirin for low-grade fevers (a really high fever would be a different story); they would be more likely to recommend hot ginger tea, hot broth, or a steam to help the body heat up and fight off the infection. Ayurveda believes that if you eat a heavy meal when your tongue is coated, you will be overloading the digestive system at a time when it can't handle it. Light, warm foods and drinks such as soups or teas, as well as pungent herbs and spices like ginger, turmeric, black pepper, cardamom, coriander, and cinnamon, are good choices when you're not feeling well because they help to rebuild the fire and clear out the *ama* that has built up and may be causing the illness. When your mother fed you tea or soup and light, dry toast for an upset stomach, she was only following the natural wisdom handed down from one generation to the next.

To get a better picture of how the ancient wisdom of Ayurveda translates into modern science, let's look at how digestion actually works.

FOLLOWING THE PATH OF DIGESTION

The simple and "healthy" digestive path leads from the mouth to the esophagus to the stomach to the small intestine to the large intestine and finally to the anus for excretion of waste material. Each step is a precursor to the next, and if any one step is not carried out efficiently, digestion will be compromised.

The first—or, in Ayurvedic terms, the Kapha—step in digestion occurs when you smell food and, in response, hunger signals your body to secrete saliva, which contains the enzyme that begins to break down carbohydrates in the mouth. In Ayurveda, food is supposed to be a sensory experience. Smell, taste, and color all help to stimulate digestion. You probably know this yourself from having passed a bakery or a restaurant with wonderful smells wafting out the door. Invariably, you say to yourself, That really smells good. I'm really hungry!

Because digestion begins in the mouth, it's important to chew your food properly (your mother was right about that, too), because if it isn't broken down enough at this early stage, your stomach will have to deal with particles that are larger than it was intended to handle.

The stomach (the end stage of Kapha digestion and beginning of Pitta digestion) secretes hydrochloric acid, which is mainly responsible for digesting protein. The contents of the stomach are then moved to the small intestine, and the pancreas begins to secrete enzymes that digest the food even further, reducing it to smaller particles and turning the acid to alkaline. At this point, nutrients will pass through the wall of the small intestine to nourish the various tissues; the remaining contents of the small intestine will pass to the large intestine, where minerals and water will be reabsorbed and the waste material will continue on the path to excretion. (This is the Vata phase of digestion.) If all goes well, you should be moving your bowels once or twice a day. Less than once or more than three times a day is not considered normal in Ayurveda and should be addressed. My clients always seem surprised when I tell them this; so many people have been living with constipation for so long that they consider it completely normal. Western practitioners are also aware of the serious problems that can result from chronic constipation, which is one of the reasons we have all been urged to add more fiber to our diet. In Ayurveda and traditional Chinese medicine, however, chronic constipation is completely unacceptable and would be treated much earlier than it generally is in the Western medical establishment.

So when digestion is running smoothly, we should be processing and eliminating our food efficiently, but there are any number of factors that can disrupt or derail digestive efficiency.

WHEN DIGESTION GOES WRONG

One of the first and most important keys to proper digestion, according to Ayurveda, is eating slowly in a quiet, peaceful setting—and that doesn't mean in front of the computer or in your car. One of my biggest challenges is convincing clients to take an actual lunch break rather than eating at their desk and working at the same time, but it's very important for proper digestion. Remember when your mother told you to stay out of the pool for thirty to forty-five minutes after eating? Well, once more it turns out she was smarter than you thought. If your body is trying to digest your lunch, you won't be swimming efficiently because your blood and nervous systems can't "focus" on two things at once, and you really could get that cramp she warned you about and drown. The same logic holds true in the office. Your digestive system and your nervous system need some quiet time to process your lunch. If you want to lose weight and avoid those three-thirty sugar cravings, you need to eat a larger lunch during the Pitta time of day (ten A.M. to two P.M.), when digestion is strongest, and a lighter dinner. And you need to allow your body to concentrate on digestion—not half on digestion and half on the computer. If you eat a decent lunch in a quiet setting, then take a short, slow, five-to-ten-minute walk (not a workout) to help your digestive system get things moving, followed by a short rest—even five minutes, just to let your nervous system calm down—you'll see how much more efficiently you work through the rest of the day. Most people have experienced this when they have a nice, leisurely Sunday brunch, but it's something that you shouldn't be saving only for the occasional Sunday. If you eat your larger meal earlier, walk a bit, and then rest a few minutes, even if it means just sitting on a bench quietly for a few minutes, you should notice an improvement in your digestion and your mental clarity during the second half of the day, and you usually won't be as hungry for dinner. This is an important key to maximizing your energy, productivity, and weight management.

Again, it's worth noting that most other cultures eat this way. Europeans, Latin Americans, and Asians all eat their larger meal at noon and take some "siesta" time before returning to work. Even farmers start their chores early in the morning, take time off at the hottest part of the day, then resume their work in the afternoon and work until close to sundown.

Another reason for eating slowly, calmly, and peacefully, as I already mentioned, is to make sure you chew your food properly. If you're in a rush—literally gulping the food down—you'll be asking your stomach to process large, undigested clumps that should already have been broken down, thus disrupting the orderly flow of the digestive process. And if the stomach is unable to do its job properly, the *ama,* or toxic material, will begin to build up, causing even greater problems down the road, including indigestion, gas, bloating, and acid reflux.

Another key to digestive health and efficiency is eating the right kinds of nutrients at the proper intervals. Enormous numbers of people suffer on a daily basis from acid reflux, commonly known as heartburn, and indigestion (which accounts for the robust health of the antacid industry). A strong Pitta, or a person in a Pitta imbalance, needs to eat enough food—and, as I explained in the previous chapter, particularly enough protein—to absorb the excess hydrochloric acid secreted in the stomach. If there isn't enough food, or if you don't eat frequently enough to balance the excess acid, it can move out of the stomach and back up into the esophagus, and you'll be popping those antacids at an alarming rate. Or you may simply be eating too many of the hot and spicy or acidic foods that aggravate the fire in your belly. Either way, antacids are not the answer; they simply mask the symptoms without discovering or correcting the cause. Ultimately, too many antacids will douse your fire completely, increasing the probability that *ama,* or toxins, will build up in your system. You don't want to kill the fire, you just want to balance it with the right foods and spices. A better idea would be to cut back on the spicy and acidic foods, make sure you are eating enough protein at the proper intervals—approximately every three to four hours, but no more frequently than every three hours (which would cause you to produce too much hydrochloric acid)—and eat your largest meal in the middle of the day, when your Pitta is at its height and your hunger is strongest.

Ayurveda would also recommend that you eat more sweet, cooling fruits to balance the fire. Dr. Rama Mishra, head physician at the Maharishi Ayur-Ved Center in Colorado Springs, which was responsible for bringing transcendental meditation to the United States, continues to reiterate: "Eat more sweet, juicy fruit to cool Pitta." A high (or extreme) Pitta, particularly in the summer, might need some watermelon, sweet peaches, berries, or (my particular favorite) limeade with a pinch of sea salt—which is also great for electrolyte replacement when it's hot and you're perspiring.

As always, balance is key, and for those Vatas and Kaphas whose digestive fires tend to need boosting in the best of circumstances, eating too little or too infrequently will cause the stomach to secrete less and less hydrochloric acid because their fire will die out. This means that the food they do eat will travel from the stomach to the small intestine without having been properly digested in the previous stage of the process, and the pancreas will not receive the signal it needs to secrete the enzymes that would allow digestion to continue. And, as we've said, inefficient digestion can lead to any number of health problems down the road.

In addition, too much processed white sugar and flour, saturated fats, and processed foods that are deficient in live enzymes and nutrients can also put too much strain on the pancreas by requiring it to secrete too much insulin, leading—as we discussed in the previous chapter—to insulin resistance, obesity, and all the other health problems that go along with it.

STRESS AND THE EMOTIONAL FACTOR

We're all aware, of course, of the many ways that stress can impact health and lead to stress-related illnesses such as ulcers, ulcerative colitis, headaches, and even skin conditions like eczema and psoriasis. In Ayurveda, however, stress and digestion are inextricably intertwined. We will discuss this in more depth in the next chapter, but for now a basic overview will do.

On the simplest level, if you are stressed, your sympathetic nervous system and adrenal glands kick into fight-or-flight mode. Your breathing will be shallow, and your mouth will become dry (meaning that you are secreting less saliva), so that you will not be able to begin the digestion of carbohydrates, which occurs in the mouth. Think about it: If you're in a life-or-death situation, digestion isn't going to be your number one priority, fight or flight is. And if you are stressed because you are overworked, overbooked, or otherwise overtaxed, your sympathetic nervous system is continuously stimulated; you'll be rushing through your meal, gulping your food, and therefore not breaking it down properly from the beginning. Owing to the combination of these two factors, your digestion will be off from the moment food enters your mouth and will, therefore, continue to be off throughout the entire process. Your body doesn't really know the difference between rushing to work in traffic to meet deadlines and running away from a lion.

Under stress, Vatas may lose their appetite and become gassy and bloated; Kaphas may become lethargic and depressed; and Pittas may become more fired up, putting them at risk for high blood pressure or ulcers.

There is an undeniable and direct correlation between weight gain and a high level of stress, blood sugar swings, and an increased craving for sweets and carbohydrates that occurs when the brain demands the serotonin boost it needs to calm itself. Fight or flight causes an increased output of adrenaline and cortisol, increased blood to the muscles, and increased glycogen and blood sugar output, which leads inevitably to a blood sugar crash, fatigue, and additional cravings for sugar and carbohydrates when it's all over.

Many people don't eat much all day when they are in emergency mode and then binge on carbs and chocolate at night when they get home and let down. There are, however, other ways to calm your nervous system without undermining your health and increasing your weight. Deep breathing and yoga, for example, stimulate your parasympathetic nervous system, which is responsible for calming you down, and can help to eliminate cravings for all those sweet, creamy, grounding foods.

WHEN WE HARBOR UNDIGESTED EMOTIONS

Ayurveda believes that in addition to undigested food, you can have undigested emotions (emotional *ama*), which will also affect your digestion. If you are harboring unresolved anger or sadness or frustration, those emotions will build up, eventually causing digestive problems.

A perfect illustration of this principle would be the case of a client who came to me because neither traditional Western medicine nor complementary medical treatment had been able to cure her persistent ulcerative colitis (an inflamed and bleeding colon), a Pitta disorder or imbalance in Ayurveda. Although she seemed quiet, soft-spoken, gentle, and generally a Kapha-type personality, when I asked her to fill out a form to determine her constitutional type, she checked off all the Pitta characteristics. As we discussed her life and work and personal relationships, I learned that she was the manager of a software sales team and that her job was putting her under a lot of stress; her relationship with her significant other was also rocky, and they argued a great deal. All in all, she was overworked, overstressed, and not sufficiently nurtured. And because she was so quiet, she kept all her emotions inside. Her illness was simply her body's way of trying to get rid of the toxic emotions that she was not expressing verbally or managing well. The real prescription for this woman was to get counseling, find another job, end her destructive relationship, and get some proper exercise—calming yoga for deep breathing and to alleviate stress, and also some boxing to get out the frustration. The point of her story, however, is to indicate how easily your health can be compromised by emotional issues that impact your digestion.

Most of us have generated some symptoms of poor digestion at one time or another, many of us have lived with them for years, but because our bodies are usually so resilient, and because most doctors don't tend to examine nutrition or digestion as an indicator of emotional distress, we are likely to ignore our body's signals far too long—until our system simply can't handle the strain any longer and we develop a full-blown disease, such as my client's ulcerative colitis.

Investigating and, ultimately, validating the connection between emotions and digestion has been the ongoing work of Dr. Candace Pert, the research professor and author of *Molecules of Emotion*. Dr. Pert has demonstrated the network of communication that exists among the brain, the endocrine system, and the immune system and states that a disintegration of the mind-body connection, or living in a state of stress, worry, or anxiety, can cause incomplete or poor digestion and, ultimately, lead to weight gain, health problems, and disease. Dr. Pert also speaks about her personal experience with Ayurveda in combination with Western medicine and believes Ayurveda to be a "scientifically valid" medical tradition.

THE BOTTOM LINE

When your digestive system is working efficiently, you should be metabolizing the nutrients you take in for optimal energy, which means that you will be burning the optimal number of calories rather than storing them as body fat, and you will be excreting toxins and waste matter efficiently before they can build up and lead to chronic health problems.

The way to do this is to learn to listen to your body and to give it what it needs before it has time to break down. Just as you wouldn't purposely let your car run out of gas so that it comes to a dead halt in the middle of the highway, you shouldn't let your digestion break down to the point where your body stops functioning.

Unfortunately, in this country, we've given up too much responsibility for maintaining our own health, and our medical system is set up to "fix things" after they've broken rather than keep them in good repair. At the risk of overusing the car analogy, I have to point out that we don't expect our car insurance company to pay because we've neglected to put in the right kind of gas, or change the oil, or even keep the tires filled, but we do expect the medical profession, and specifically our health insurance company, to pay for the neglect of our bodies—for which we are really responsible. Having spent the past five years incorporating Ayurveda into my practice, I've come to realize just how out of touch with their bodies most people are. My goal is to help you to "tune in" so you will be able to lose weight, balance your cravings, and maximize both your health and your energy. In the last several years the number of visits Americans make to complementary practitioners has grown exponentially. Research has shown there were actually more visits to integrative medical practitioners than allopathic (traditional Western) practitioners in the last few years. Hopefully this means that we are all becoming more aware of the need to develop a system whereby the client, the practitioner, and the insurance companies work together to emphasize prevention and keep people healthy. It should be a team effort.

By now you should be able to understand why an imbalance of Vata, Pitta, or Kapha, eating the wrong ratios of proteins, fats, and carbohydrates, or living with chronic stress can cause digestive problems that lead to cravings, undermine your health, and cause you to gain weight.

In the next chapter we'll be discussing the ways that overconsumption of specific foods—even so-called healthy foods—can lead to serious digestive problems, especially if they are the wrong foods for your constitutional type, your ethnic heritage, or your genetic makeup. And we will talk about lifestyle issues, including our overreliance on antibiotics, that can compromise our digestion, immunity to illness, and overall health.

CHAPTER FIVE

Food Sensitivities, Blood Type, Cultural Background, and Their Relation to Cravings and Digestion

In the world of complementary medicine, traditional Chinese medicine, and Ayurveda, digestion, as I've just explained, is the key to good health. If your digestion is "off," as discussed in the previous chapter, your body's entire energy system will be functioning at less than optimum level. In this chapter I'm going to explain some of the factors that may compromise your digestion and offer some ideas that should help you take charge of your own destiny by increasing your energy levels and improving your overall health.

Before we go any further, however, I'd like to help you determine whether there are any foods or lifestyle issues that might be keeping you from achieving maximum digestive health. Please take the time to answer the following questions and see if you notice any patterns developing.

As you read through the rest of the chapter, keep your answers in mind. You should begin to see how they provide clues to the foods that might be upsetting your digestion, compromising your weight, creating unhealthy cravings, and, ultimately, undermining your general good health. They should also help to determine whether your stress levels are pushing you to exhaustion and increasing your need for foods that will ground and calm you.

THE FOOD SENSITIVITIES QUESTIONNAIRE

DIGESTION

Use the numbers to indicate how often you experience these digestive conditions.

1 = All the time/daily
2 = 1–2/week
3 = Occasionally
4 = Hardly ever
5 = Never

__ Burping and belching?

__ Gas?

__ Bloating?

__ Constipation?

__ Diarrhea/loose bowels?

Have you ever taken antibiotics (even as a child) for a specific ailment such as earaches or to clear up acne?   Yes   No

Did you take acidophilus/probiotics (good bacteria) after you finished the antibiotics?   Yes   No

Have you ever been told you could possibly have candida, yeast, or parasites?   Yes   No

Do you crave sweet foods or carbohydrates?   Yes   No

If you indulge in sweet foods, do you have any side effects or reactions, such as gas, bloating, or fatigue? What reactions, if any? _____

What types of cravings do you have? _____

BLOOD TYPE AND CULTURAL BACKGROUND

What blood type are you?* _____

From what culture or cultures did your family originate? _____

> * If you do not know your blood type, first call your physician. He or she may well have it on record. Otherwise, there are inexpensive and reliable home blood-typing kits, such as those distributed by North American Pharmacal and by Eldoncard, that will provide the answer. They are available without a prescription and can be found in some drugstores. Or you can find more information on our Web site at www.thebalancedapproach.com

THE FOOD SENSITIVITIES QUESTIONNAIRE (continued)

Do you feel better or prefer eating as a (check one):

Vegan (no animal products)? ___

Vegetarian (lacto-ovo: eats eggs and dairy products, but no fish, meat, or poultry)? ___

Non–meat eater (does not eat meat or poultry, but eats eggs, dairy, and fish)? ___

Meat eater (feels best when eating chicken, turkey, and/or red meat)? ___

ACTIVITY LEVEL (TOO MUCH OR TOO LITTLE?)

Do you exercise? ___

How many times per week? ___

For how long? ___

What is your favorite activity? _____

Do you have variety or do you do the same workout all the time? _____

HOW MANY TIMES PER DAY OR WEEK DO YOU EAT:

Whole-wheat products: cereal, bread, pasta, cookies, crackers, etc.? ___

Cow's milk dairy products: milk, yogurt, cheese, ice cream, frozen yogurt, whey protein powders? ___

Soy products: tofu, tempeh, protein powders, vegetable burgers, soy substitutes? ___

Chicken? ___

Peanuts/peanut butter? ___

Warm foods such as soups and cooked vegetables? ___

Cold foods such as raw vegetables and cold cereals? ___

Olive oil? ___

Flaxseed oil/fish oils? ___

Any essential fatty acid? ___

Saturated fats? ___

SLEEP/ENERGY LEVEL

Do you need to set the alarm to wake up in the morning?   Yes   No

How many hours would you sleep if you didn't set the alarm? ___

Do you often wake up feeling tired?   Yes   No

THE FOOD SENSITIVITIES QUESTIONNAIRE (continued)

Do you experience blood sugar swings throughout the day (i.e., lightheaded, dizzy, low energy)?	Yes	No
Do you find yourself craving sugar, coffee, or Coke during the day or around three to five P.M.?	Yes	No
Do you need coffee or Coke to get going in the morning?	Yes	No
Do you find it difficult to wind down in the evening to fall asleep?	Yes	No

STRESS LEVEL

On a scale of 1 to 10, how would you rate your stress:

At home? ___

At work? ___

ALLERGIES AND FOOD SENSITIVITIES

Practitioners of complementary medicine who have come out of the traditional Western medical establishment, including Dr. James Braly, M.D., author of *Dr. Braly's Food Allergy and Nutrition Revolution,* Dr. Andrew Weil, M.D., author of *Eight Weeks to Optimum Health,* and Jeffrey Bland, Ph.D., founder of The Institute for Functional Medicine and one of the top nutritional biochemists in the country, all recognize the effects that nutrition, digestion, food allergies, and sensitivities can have on a variety of health problems, ranging from irritable bowel syndrome to attention deficit disorder to arthritis, migraines, and weight management.

Although it might be a "stretch" for you, at this point, to see the relationship between your digestion and this wide range of seemingly unrelated ailments, I've seen my clients improve over and over again simply by changing their diet. If you consider the fact that all the systems in your body are interconnected, and that a failure in one system will necessarily affect all the others, the reason for such improvement shouldn't be too difficult to understand. Your digestive system is connected to your adrenal glands, which are connected to your immune system, your endocrine system, and so on, and these systems can affect your metabolism, and every other system that is intended to keep your body in balance. Dr. Bland constantly refers to this as a "weblike connection," and Dr. Pert, as we've already discussed, has been instrumental in proving scientifically and explaining the mind-body connection. So, once again, it makes sense that if you eat something that irritates or disturbs your digestion, it will have an impact on the rest of your body. And if you have the same neurotransmitters in your brain that you have in your gut, it makes sense to assume that if your digestion is "off," your brain will also be less alert and clear.

Allergies

Allergies, whether to foods, airborne pollens, or other irritants, have long been recognized in Western medicine as serious and potentially life-threatening health concerns. If you're allergic to something, you usually know it because you experience an almost immediate reaction. Your immune system mobilizes IgE (immunoglobin E) antibodies—proteins that naturally exist in the blood—to combat the foreign invader, and you sneeze, or you become congested, or your eyes become itchy and watery, or you develop hives. Your body is trying to localize and get rid of the foreign substance. In the worst-case scenario, when an allergy is extremely severe, you could go into anaphylactic shock, your throat might close up, or your tongue might swell, creating a life-or-death emergency. We've all heard about children, for example, who are highly allergic to peanuts or about people who can have a fatal reaction to bee stings. And if you've ever had a positive reaction to a skin-prick allergy test, you'll remember the redness and swelling at the site of the prick that was caused by IgE antibodies responding to the allergen. In fact, one potential danger of genetically engineered foods is that we can no longer tell whether there might not be, for example, a peanut gene crossed with a soybean, which could pose a serious risk for people who are allergic to peanuts.

There is, however, a different kind of reaction, not so widely recognized among Western medical practitioners, that may be making you miserable, compromising your health and energy, and preventing you from maintaining optimal weight without your even realizing it.

Sensitivities

You may have a "sensitivity" to a particular food that is not the same thing as a full-blown allergy. Food sensitivities cause your immune system to send out different kinds of antibodies, which are referred to as IgG, IgA, and IgM, among others. Your reaction to these antibodies can be delayed anywhere from one hour to as long as three to four days (which is about how long it can take the food you eat today to be cleared from your system). Because of this delay, you may not always recognize the association between the reaction and its cause. You may feel bloated or have gas, you may have a headache, your joints could swell or become inflamed, or you might develop any number of other uncomfortable but not necessarily acute symptoms that are not readily identified as resulting from the food you ate.

If you break out in hives every time you eat a strawberry, you may, quite logically, decide that the pleasure simply isn't worth the pain. But if you eat a bowl of pasta, for example, and three days later experience lethargy, gas and bloating, or congestion and sinus problems, you may never even recognize that the wheat or gluten in the pasta was the source of your pain. And if this has been happening to you regularly for a period of years, you may just begin to think it's normal. But, as I've said before, it isn't. Rather, it's a sign that your body is trying to defend itself against the alien irritant and is therefore unable to do its digestive work properly.

If the irritation goes on long enough (and for many people it probably started as far back as infancy or childhood), your colon can develop tiny tears, a condition known as "leaky gut," that will allow undigested food particles to enter the bloodstream. Once these undigested particles (or *ama,* in Ayurvedic terms) are transported by the bloodstream to the tissues, they can cause inflammation, irritation, and pain. And their presence will prevent your body from working with optimum efficiency because your immune system will be stressed from having to fight off the foreign invaders. So once again, it seems clear and logical that digestion would have a significant effect on overall health.

BUT I THOUGHT IT WAS GOOD FOR ME!

You may, in fact, have been overconsuming some of these foods just because you've been told they were "healthy" for you. A good example would be whole-wheat bread, oatmeal, or bran cereal. It's true that these grains contain the fiber that the medical profession has been telling us we need in our diet. The problem is that many of these grains also contain gluten, to which many people are known to be allergic or sensitive, and which may actually have been creating toxins in your system because you have not been digesting it properly. Irritable bowel syndrome, Crohn's disease, and colitis, for example, can all be related to gluten sensitivity. I'll be talking in greater detail about overuse of gluten later in this chapter. Suffice it to say for now that even the healthiest foods can be detrimental to health and digestion if you are consuming them in excess.

Continuing to eat foods you don't digest properly—even if you think they're healthy—can cause your metabolism to work less effectively. Your digestive fire can become less efficient, and instead of burning nutrients to expend as energy, you will start to store them as body fat or *ama*. In the end, it always comes down to the same thing—eating the foods that are right for you in order to keep digestion strong and thus maximize your health and control your weight. Not until I began to study Ayurveda did I really understand that broccoli isn't always good for everyone and chocolate isn't necessarily bad, but that it's really a question of whether or not you can digest it, how often you eat it, how it is prepared, and whether it's appropriate for your own constitutional needs.

Look back at your answers to the questionnaire (page 84) and see if there are foods you've been eating over and over again. Then try to keep a food journal, jotting down what you've eaten each day and how you feel afterward, both physically and emotionally. Before too long you should have a clear indication of how much repetition there is in your diet, and if you've not been feeling well, it might be a sign that the foods you've been overconsuming are having a negative effect on your overall well-being.

DIGESTION, IMMUNITY, AND FOOD SENSITIVITIES

How well we are able to tolerate or fight off the effects of foods to which we might be sensitive can depend on how healthy we are to begin with or, to put it another way, on the strength of our immune system. In Ayurveda, the word *ojas* is used to describe immunity, while *prana* is the term for life force, both your own and the life force in the foods you eat. And, as I've been saying all along, Ayurveda believes that food should be not only immune system enhancing, but also nurturing and strengthening to your life force. Food itself should also have *prana,* which will help to strengthen the body's own life force; but if you eat nothing but dead, overprocessed foods that are far removed from their own original "life," they will have less nutritional value and will even detract from the efficiency of your immune system by forcing you to work harder to digest them. Think about the difference between a carrot grown in organic soil that's rich in minerals and pulled straight from the ground. Now think of canned string beans that may have been on the grocer's shelf for months. The string beans will be pale green and tasteless, while the carrot will be vibrant with flavor to stimulate your digestive fire. Obviously the carrot will also have more *prana,* or life force, not to mention a higher nutrient content.

Ideally, a well-nourished, healthy baby born to a well-nourished mother looks all pink and radiant and chubby (the baby, that is). That baby is full of strong *ojas* and is dependent on its mother to strengthen its immune system during the first six weeks to six months of life. Unfortunately for many of us, however, the immune system probably began to be compromised at a very early age. Research now indicates that a healthy baby, born to a healthy mother, who is breast-fed for *at least* the first six weeks of life (and preferably the first six months to one year), will have better immunity than one who is not breast-fed, or who is breast-fed by an unhealthy or malnourished mother. According to an article published in *Mothering* magazine, one study published in the *Journal of the National Cancer Institute* showed that babies who are breast-fed for at least one month are 21 percent less likely to develop childhood acute leukemia; and another study, conducted in Australia, showed that babies who were not exclusively breast-fed were 27 percent more likely to develop asthma by age six. So a healthy, well-nourished mother with strong *ojas* and *prana* can pass that along to her baby. The mom needs to make sure she maintains her own strength and health during pregnancy and nursing.

The Antibiotic Story

But if that healthy baby, however he or she was originally nourished, begins to develop the earaches or strep throats that are so common in the early years (or Kapha time), a pediatrician will most likely treat the infection with antibiotics. We all harbor millions of "good" bacteria in our colon at all times, and those good bacteria help us to digest our food, protect us from invasive "bad" bacteria, and keep us in good health. When a baby (or an adult, for that matter) is given an antibiotic, the drug will certainly clear up the infection by killing the bad bacteria that caused it, but it will also kill off some of the good bacteria that are necessary for maintaining immunity. If the digestive system was already compromised by less than optimal nourishment, and if the infections recur, more antibiotics will usually be prescribed, which will continue to kill off more good bacteria with the bad and further compromise the digestive tract and the immune system.

Along with the millions of both beneficial and harmful bacteria in our system, all of us also harbor in our intestinal tract a form of yeast called *Candida albicans*. The bacteria and yeast, under optimum conditions, live in a symbiotic balance with one another. If the bacteria are constantly diminished by too many antibiotics, the yeast has a chance to overgrow, leading to a condition known as candidiasis, the fungal form of candida. The yeast can flourish to the point where, eventually, it can break down the lining of the gastrointestinal tract— a condition, as we've mentioned, known as "leaky gut"—releasing allergens and toxins into the bloodstream, where they can produce any number of unpleasant symptoms, from gas and bloating to constipation or diarrhea, headaches, irritated or inflamed joints, weight gain, even hepatitis, PMS, or depression, weakening the immune system even further.

If you're a baker, you'll know that if you dissolve yeast in warm water and add sugar, the yeast will burble up and your baked goods will rise. Baker's yeast and candida, I hasten to point out, are two different species of yeast, but I think the comparison provides a useful visual image for what happens in your colon when the candida gets out of control. An overgrowth of the organism, even before it causes leaky gut, can lead to fatigue, mental fuzziness, attention deficit problems, weight gain, depression, and further cravings for sugar and carbohydrates.

It's time to look again at the answers you gave to the questionnaire. If you were not breast-fed or if you suffered from repeated infections as a child and were given antibiotics, you may well be harboring an overgrowth of yeast that is weighing you down. A practitioner versed in complementary medicine would understand the importance of following up a prescription for antibiotics with a course of probiotics to return good bacteria and rebalance the microflora in the digestive tract. Unfortunately, most traditional Western physicians don't generally know to prescribe probiotics for their patients, probably because they have very little training in digestion and nutrition. In chapter 8 I'll not only suggest ways to gently cleanse the buildup of yeast and other toxins from your system, I'll also offer you ways to rebuild the good bacteria that will help to increase your immunity.

Stress, Adrenal Health, and Immunity

As I started to talk about in the previous chapter, when we reach adulthood, we put more environmental, work-related, and other stresses on our immune system. If, on top of this daily stress, we continue to eat foods we can't digest properly, our *ojas,* or immune system, can be severely compromised and we can increase the chances of exacerbating some type of health problem. According to complementary medicine, each of us has some weak spot, or weak link in the chain, and when we become exhausted or depleted, some problem will usually kick up. For one person it could be simply a cold. For someone else it could be asthma, irritable bowel syndrome, headaches, arthritis, or some other problem.

One of the keys to our ability to fight off infection and maintain strong *ojas* is the health of our adrenal glands. The adrenal glands, situated above the kidneys, are two little hormone factories. They secrete the hormones adrenaline and cortisol, which among other functions affect the body's use and digestion of all three macronutrients—proteins, fats, and carbohydrates. They also secrete the hormone corticosterone, which suppresses inflammatory reactions and affects the immune system. And finally, they manufacture and deploy epinephrine and norepinephrine, which affect heart rate and blood flow to the brain, helping us to cope with physical and emotional stress. Your sympathetic nervous system kicks in in emergencies to get you out of there. Your parasympathetic nervous system will help calm you back down when the emergency is over. Short, shallow breathing kicks off the sympathetic and signals stress; deep, relaxed breathing stimulates the parasympathetic to signal calmness and centeredness.

That's why yoga or deep breathing can be so beneficial to your health, well being, and management of stress and food cravings.

Everyone understands fight or flight. If you're walking in a parking lot at night and a mugger comes up behind you, you'll go into fight or flight. It's how mothers pick up cars off children. And at a time like that, as we've already explained, digestion will not be your body's highest priority. Your sympathetic nervous system was designed to "shoot out" adrenaline in an emergency—for a short period of time. But if we live a constantly fast-paced, high-stress lifestyle, as so many of us do, we go into prolonged adrenal overload, which can eventually compromise the immune system and lead to poor energy, bad digestion, and weight gain.

So the adrenal glands really have two functions that are vital to our health—they help us to fight off infection, and they are vital to our management of stress. Sad to say, most of us have been pushing our adrenal glands to do more than they can manage all at the same time. If you consistently eat foods that compromise your digestion and hence your immunity, your adrenals and digestive system will be working overtime to keep you healthy. And if, on top of that, you are constantly stressed—as so many of us are—you'll also be asking these same glands to handle a perpetual state of fight or flight. Sooner or later they will simply be depleted—or "shot," as we say in the trade.

If your job has you working in overdrive, if your personal life is stressful, if you're fighting traffic, noise, and conflicting commitments and you never take a vacation, you are definitely in fight-or-flight mode. If you're a Vata personality type, your problem will be even greater, because Vatas tend to be scattered and stressed out even at the best of times. You may find yourself craving lots of creamy, sweet foods to calm and ground you, and might need a caffeine or sugar pick-me-up at three or four o'clock every afternoon because your adrenal glands are exhausted, Vata'd out, and are running out of steam.

Now that your immune system is compromised by stress, and exacerbated by your constantly eating too many of the foods to which you are sensitive, you may notice a flare-up of symptoms in whatever happens to be your weakest point. For some people it might be stomach disorders, for others headaches or sinus infections or arthritis pain. If your *ojas,* or immune system, were really strong, you might not experience symptoms because your body would be able to fight off the effects of the irritant; but if you're overstressed, overtired, or overworked, you'll begin to notice them. Many people, for example, seem to have a tendency to develop canker sores. If they're well rested, eating well, and exercising, the canker sores don't flare up; when they do get one, it's a signal to recoup because they've been pushing themselves too far. These symptoms are manifestations of a problem that has been brewing for a while.

One of the first steps to take toward regaining your balance, your immunity, and your digestive health is to determine which of the foods you've been eating might be responsible for causing your distress.

What Determines My Food Sensitivities?

Any number of factors can determine the specific foods to which a person is sensitive, and which foods he or she does or does not digest well, but one of the key determinants may be related to cultural, ethnic, or ancestral background.

Ayurveda talks about a diet based on the theory of the three constitutional body types; in *The Metabolic Typing Diet,* William L. Wolcott talks about eating according to your particular metabolic type; and Peter J. D'Adamo, N.D., in *Eat Right for Your Type,* as mentioned earlier, advocates foods that are appropriate for your blood type. These books and many others, such as *Your Hidden Food Allergies Are Making You Fat,* by Rudy Rivera and Roger D. Deutsch, are all, to some degree, advocating a diet based on your individual biochemistry, constitutional type, and genetic heritage.

Cultural Diversity and Genetic Background

Most of us have heard about the "healthy" Asian diet, based mainly on soy, fish, vegetables and nongluten grains like rice, with very little meat or poultry, and about the fact that Asians have a very low rate of heart disease—until they come to the United States and adopt an American diet. The implication, of course, is that the Asian diet is healthy while the American diet is not. The missing piece of this equation is the question "Healthy for whom?" Just because the Asian diet appears to be healthy for Asians does not mean it would be equally healthy for people of all other cultural and genetic backgrounds. In fact, a large percentage of the Asian population is lactose intolerant. Dairy products do not constitute a significant percentage of the Asian diet, and as a consequence of their genetic heritage, many Asians are lacking the enzyme that would allow them to digest large quantities of dairy products. On the other hand, the descendants of people who lived in populations that were dependent on the herding of sheep or goats often produce lactose as adults and digest dairy products well. Having ancestors from Europe, the Middle East, India, or East Africa increases the probability that organic dairy products may be your best source of protein. But that diet, too, might be inappropriate for people of many other cultures.

Lactose intolerance, which is caused by the lack of a particular digestive enzyme, is not the same thing as an allergy or food sensitivity, which triggers the deployment of antibodies into the bloodstream; but it is a useful way of indicating that the foods on which the people of one culture thrive might be the very foods that would make those of another culture ill. If you lack the enzyme to digest lactose, you will have trouble digesting milk products, which means you could be subject to gas, bloating, or diarrhea. In Ayurveda, the key is to not eat what you can't digest.

Oldways Preservation and Exchange Trust is a nonprofit, Boston-based organization that has been researching the ancestral diets of various native populations and has published a series of "food pyramids" for each of these groups. In part 2 of this book, we'll be talking more about various ethnic food pyramids and how they can help you to diversify and, in effect, "spice up" your own meals with healthy, well-flavored foods. For now, it's enough for you to understand that there is no "one size fits all" diet that works for everyone and that one of the ways to determine what is appropriate for any individual would be to look at that person's ancestral, cultural, or ethnic heritage. Even the American Dietetic Association is now acknowledging that it's important to consider the diets of various ethnic cultures rather than recommending the same "standard American diet" for everyone.

The Blood Type Factor

Peter D'Adamo, as I've said, approaches the issue of ethnic diets and food sensitivities by looking at individual blood types. While critics have questioned the "science" underlying the correlation between A, B, O typing and food sensitivities, logically it might make sense when you consider that many people who share a cultural background also share the same blood type, and different blood types contain different antigens. There are actually thousands of different antigens on the surface of red blood cells, but one type of antigen, the A, B, O system, dictates blood transfusion compatibility.

Of the four types (O, A, B, and AB), type O (the oldest, or original, blood type) is the universal donor and type AB (the newest of the types) is the universal recipient. Beyond these exceptions, however, if a person of one blood type were to be given a transfusion of another type, the antigens in the recipient's blood would create antibodies to fight off the invader, and as a result, the recipient's blood would clot up, or agglutinate to try to protect the body from allowing the invader into their system. Think of it as one type of blood being "allergic" to all the other types.

D'Adamo postulates that, to a less extreme degree, the same thing happens when a person continuously eats foods that are inappropriate for his or her particular blood type. An excess of incompatible foods in the system will cause chronic agglutination, or "clumping up," as your body tries to rid itself of the perceived toxic substances. Proteins, called lectins, that are present in the liver and kidneys will stick to the perceived toxins in order to surround them with a mucous substance and carry them out of the system. This would be comparable, in Ayurveda, to what happens when too much *ama*—indigestible or toxic food particles—collects in the intestine and has to be expelled. The person probably won't have an extreme or life-threatening reaction, but he or she will experience various digestive disorders and will feel clogged up and congested.

According to D'Adamo's theory, type Os, the oldest, original blood type, were originally hunter-gatherers, designed with stronger stomach acids that allowed them to break down and digest animal proteins; type Bs are of nomadic backgrounds and are adapted to digest beef, goat, sheep, and dairy products but don't do well on farm animals like chicken. Type As evolved with agricultural development; their stomach acids are not as strong as those of either the hunter-gatherers or the nomads, and therefore they don't do well with the heavier meat proteins; and ABs combine the genetics of both the nomadic and agricultural types and, therefore, do best on a mixed diet.

I like to ask clients if they know their blood type just to compare it to their stated food preferences.

One example, taken from my personal experience, involves a client of the Balanced Approach who is of Brazilian background. Before she moved to the United States from her native country, she was lean and trim, but after living here for a while she began to develop digestive problems, gained weight, and noticed that her energy levels had dropped. When we compared the diet she had eaten in Brazil with the foods she was consuming in this country, the answers became clear rather quickly. Brazilians eat quite a bit more beef than most Americans, but their beef cattle are free range and therefore lean and chemical free. Brazilians also consume more fish, dark green leafy vegetables, oils, good EFAs, and flavorful condiments than she was eating here. The quality of her food dropped here and she was eating a lot more processed foods and gluten grains. When she went back to eating organic meats (which are readily available even in most supermarkets), more vegetables, and more oils and spices, her digestive problems quickly disappeared and her energy levels returned to normal. This is not only a clear example of how digestion is, more often than not, the key to good health, but also indicates that eating a diet not compatible with our cultural (and therefore constitutional) background can have a significant effect on our overall well-being.

It should be said that not all ethnic or ancestral diets are equally healthy, and a diet that is heavily dependent on beef may not be the best choice for your health, but if you're going to be "carnivorous" come what may, trying to find organic, free-range beef is still the best choice.

DISCOVERING YOUR OWN SENSITIVITIES

Understandably, it is not so easy for most of us in the American melting pot to determine our specific cultural heritage. We might be part Scotch-Irish and part German, or part Italian and part Eastern European, or an even more complicated cultural mix. But if you think about the foods you consume consistently in large quantities and about the way you feel after you eat them, you should be able to determine those foods that simply do not agree with you. To put it another way, you should be able to pinpoint your food sensitivities. If you look back to the answers you gave to the questionnaire (page 84), you may already be gathering some clues to your own sensitivities.

VARIETY AND BALANCE

Whether or not we agree that blood type is the key to determining food sensitivities—and it would certainly appear from my own experience with clients who have profited from following D'Adamo's diet that this is at least an interesting variable to consider—one certain answer to overcoming their effects is to eat a wide variety of foods rather than the same ones over and over again.

One of the problems with the average American diet is that we tend to overconsume a limited number of foods over an extended period of time. Not only can this lead to cravings for the tastes and qualities of foods you've been denying yourself (because eating bland, boring foods is simply not satisfying), but it can also mean that you might be increasing, or even creating, sensitivities to those foods you overconsume. The lack of dietary variety is key to many of the chronic health problems we experience in this country.

In the best of all possible worlds, it would no doubt be wise never to eat any food you don't digest well, because if you aren't digesting a food properly, toxins will build up in your system even before you start feeling discomfort or pain. In the real world, however, it's difficult to avoid many foods entirely, and even though you may have a cultural or genetic sensitivity to a particular food, if you eat it no more than once every four to five days, you will probably be able to tolerate it without too much problem because you will not be placing too much strain on your intestinal tract. The traditional "rotation" diet is about avoiding the same foods and families of foods for a four-day period. It doesn't mean you can never have them, you just need to rotate. I can eat pizza or ice cream once in a while without any problem, but if I ate pizza every day for five days, my stomach would hurt, my skin would break out, and I wouldn't be happy. If you eat the same thing over and over again, and if it is something to which you are sensitive, you will potentially cause all kinds of digestive difficulties. As I've said, it takes about three to four days for the foods we eat to travel through and be eliminated from our digestive tract, and health problems can arise when we don't allow ourselves enough time to clear the irritant from our system. Going back to Dr. D'Adamo's blood type theory, even too much chicken, the animal protein of choice for millions of fat-conscious Americans, may cause serious digestive problems for people with B-type blood, who are not genetically adapted to digest chicken well.

However healthy a particular food might be, if it doesn't agree with *you,* and if you eat it too often, you may be jeopardizing not only your physical health, but also your mental and emotional health. Even broccoli, if it causes bloating and gas, isn't a healthy food for you to consume in large quantities. I suppose you could call this a variation on the theme of "too much of a good thing . . . is not a good thing."

WHEAT, GLUTEN, DAIRY, AND SOY: THE MAJOR CULPRITS

For Americans, the primary culprits seem to be wheat, gluten, dairy, and soy, as well as peanuts and sometimes corn. If you are among those who are sensitive to one or more of these foods, and if you consume them too often, you may be subject to symptoms ranging from gas and bloating to constipation or diarrhea to fatigue, low energy, depression, and dark circles under your eyes. Gluten is the protein fraction that is responsible for allowing wheat, oats, rye, barley, spelt, and kamut—grains that are the most popular in this country— to "stick together" and form a dough. Unfortunately, as I've said, because we have been consistently urged to "get more fiber" in our diet, most Americans are now overconsuming wheat and gluten products.

The obvious answer, and the one I've been urging throughout this book, is to incorporate more nongluten grains—millet, buckwheat, quinoa, amaranth, and corn—as well as brown rice and sweet and white potatoes into our diet. Nongluten flours, grains, breads, cookies, and crackers are all readily available, and by rotating the kinds of grains and starches we consume, we avoid overloading the colon with foods that are difficult to digest or to which we might be sensitive, and we encourage our system to more efficiently process the nutrients we do consume. So if you are a Vata, who can handle more starchy carbohydrates than a Pitta or Kapha, apple-shaped person who holds abdominal fat and is trying to "trim down," you might want to have sweet potato one day, basmati rice the next, and corn the third.

In addition, no matter who you are, the two virtually foolproof and healthy ways to add fiber and nonstarchy carbohydrates to your diet without exacerbating food sensitivities are, first of all, to eat fewer processed foods and, second, to eat more fresh fruits and vegetables. If you haven't figured it out already, "Eat your vegetables" is definitely my mantra—and once again, this is a recommendation on which the American Dietetic Association, the American Heart Association, and the fitness world (including hard-core bodybuilders) agree. Vegetables, properly prepared for your constitutional type with spices and oils, are one food that almost everyone digests well and that do not create the elevated insulin levels caused by consuming heavier or more refined carbohydrates. The more carbohydrates we obtain from leafy green vegetables, the less likely we are to be subject to the blood sugar swings that create our cravings for sweets. And remember, because greens are *bitter*, they also help to cut body fat and aid digestion—not to mention their powerful antioxidant properties. But despite almost universal agreement among all branches of health practitioners about the health and nutritional benefits to be derived from eating fruits and vegetables, a study published in the *American Journal of Public Health* indicates that only 9 percent of Americans eat five servings of fruits and vegetables each day, 45 percent eat no fruit at all, and 22 percent eat no vegetables. In part 2, I'm going to be giving you many recipes and suggestions for incorporating more vegetables into your diet by preparing them in ways that make them taste better than you've ever imagined vegetables could be.

While wheat and gluten may be the biggest culprits in this country when it comes to food sensitivities, there are certainly others. One of these, despite its many health benefits, is soy. For a variety of reasons, many Americans are now consuming *too much* soy in many forms that are hard to digest, and as I hope I've helped you to understand by now, it is definitely possible to consume too much even of a good thing.

Many people, quite logically, have dealt with their lactose intolerance by drinking soy milk, eating soy cheese, and switching from ice cream to tofu-based frozen desserts. And many women have added a lot of soy to their diets for cancer prevention. But the problem again is that, *in excess,* soy can also be irritating to the intestinal tract.

Studies have indicated that many Caucasians don't digest soy very well. As it happens, I can tell you from personal experience that eating too much soy can be problematic for some people, because that's exactly what happened to me. After I read *Eat Right for Your Type,* and knowing I have type A blood, I realized there might be a correlation between my blood type and the fact that I had never done well eating large quantities of meat. At about the same time, for ethical reasons, I decided to make a serious effort to follow a vegan diet, which meant eating no animal products at all—not only no meat, fish, or poultry, but no cheese and no dairy. I bought soy milk and soy protein powder and used tofu as my main protein source. About three months into the diet, I started to experience serious pain in my lower abdomen—sometimes so bad that I was literally doubled over. After a while, I began to realize that whenever I experienced the pain, I absolutely could not even look at a soy product. Somehow it had simply never occurred to me that I was overdosing on soy and had developed terrible gas pains. When I stopped eating soy for a few days, the pain subsided. And when, sometime later, I slowly began to reintroduce it into my diet, I found I could tolerate it once every four or five days, but no more frequently. By overconsuming this theoretically healthy food, I had created a sensitivity to it and irritated my intestinal tract (although many of my Caucasian Vegan friends use it as their staple protein with no digestive problems at all). Since I'm Caucasian, not East Asian, it makes sense that soy would not have been a staple of my ancestral diet; Asians themselves don't consume it in the quantities or in the indigestible forms I had been eating, and Asian cooking always includes digestive herbs and spices such as ginger. Ayurveda would no doubt suggest that I never eat soy again, and as a nutritionist, I should have known better than to fall prey to the "more must be better" American philosophy. But I can, as it happens, digest miso soup and *edamame* (Japanese soybeans) more frequently than other, more concentrated, synthetic soy products. As an addendum to my personal soy saga, I should remind you that just because we call it tofu, and it comes in cubes, as ice cream, or disguised as a burger, soy is a *bean,* and those constitutional types who need to stay away from airy, gas-inducing foods ought to be particularly careful about the quantities of soy in their diet and pay attention to how it is prepared.

The Bottom Line

There are a few easy ways to figure out which foods are causing your particular digestive problems. First, determine your symptoms. Gas and bloating, for example, are not normal (unless you are a Vata or in a Vata imbalance, and even then, following a diet that is appropriate for your constitutional type will significantly reduce your symptoms), so if you experience these symptoms on a regular basis, try to determine what you have eaten that may be causing them. Are you eating the same foods over and over again? Try to expand your repertoire. Alternate wheat-based foods with those made from quinoa, corn, buckwheat, or other flours; look for cow's milk alternatives; cut back on your tofu habit. Simply by *varying* your diet, you will probably feel better, digest your food more efficiently, and get rid of those annoying, if not debilitating, symptoms you have thought you'd be living with forever. In the fitness business, I see both clients and professionals who are living on whey protein shakes and protein bars and who have gas and bloating problems all the time.

In general, the more pure, whole foods we eat, the better off we will be. Not only do processed foods often contain hidden ingredients such as peanuts, corn, soy, wheat, or dairy that are likely to kick off one kind of sensitivity or another, but they do not contain enough live enzymes to create good bacteria in the colon to help fight off disease. Learning how to add rotation and variety to your diet and to use "fast foods" like protein bars only when necessary can improve digestion, energy, and weight loss. "Fake foods" are not meant to be lived on. The body knows the difference.

By eating a wide variety of clean, nutritious, fresh foods, you will avoid overloading your digestive tract, and thus your immune system, with any one food to which you might be sensitive. You will also get more pleasure out of what you're eating because it will taste better and you won't be suffering the unpleasant aftereffects you may have come to think of as normal.

CHAPTER SIX

Strength in Balance

How to Increase Lean Muscle, Burn Fat, and Relieve Stress Through Exercise, with a Special Emphasis on the Balancing Powers of Yoga

Balance is the all-important factor in a fighter's attitude or stance. Without balance at all times, he can never be effective.

BRUCE LEE, *The Tao of Jeet Kune Do*

In the previous chapters, we've been talking about how you can curb your cravings by eating foods that are appropriate for your body type, thereby optimizing your digestive health and efficiency. The one remaining component of any health and fitness program has only been touched on in passing, and that, of course, is exercise.

Right now, I can hear the pages turning as you flip to the next chapter, thinking, Well, I know I should exercise, but I'll just get my diet in order first and worry about the exercise part later. The problem is that food and diet are only half the equation. With all the medical and media emphasis on the subject in recent years, it would be almost impossible for anyone not to be aware of how important exercise is for good health and weight management. Yet according to the Surgeon General's 1996 *Report on Physical Activity and Health,* 24 percent of Americans do no form of leisure-time physical activity, and 54 percent do less than the recommended minimum of thirty minutes of moderate activity on most days, leaving only 22 percent of adults who are physically active for at least half an hour a day. The International Dance and Exercise Association reports similar statistics in their November/December 2000 publication: "It is estimated that only about 20 percent of Americans meet the Centers for Disease Control and Prevention/American College of Sports Medicine recommendations for physical activity and 25 percent are not active at all. More than 250,000 deaths per year due to all causes are attributed to a sedentary lifestyle." To make matters worse, it appears that our children may be less fit than ever as well. While the Centers for Disease Control and Prevention suggest that the goal for elementary school children should be thirty to sixty minutes of physical activity per day, one in every four children receives no physical education in school, and the average child from the age of six to eleven watches about twenty-five hours of television a week. As a result, approximately 10 percent of America's children are now obese.

Although lack of time is certainly an issue for many people, I believe one of the most significant reasons for the discrepancy between what we know and what we do is basically the same as the reason most people find it impossible to comply with any restrictive diet for an extended period of time. Just as there is no perfect, "one size fits all" diet, there is no one exercise program that will be appropriate or effective for all people. And if something—be it diet or exercise—doesn't produce results or isn't enjoyable, no one is going to stick with it.

Another reason is the quintessentially American all-or-nothing approach to so many things we do. Too many people think that if they can't work out every day, there's no point even in starting. I hope to show you that this simply isn't true, that you can "start small" and not be overwhelmed. If you do that, you will see results, and you will want to stick with your program because it feels right, not because you are obligated.

Getting started always seems to be the hardest part of any program. As you know by now, six to ten A.M. is the Kapha time of day, so it is actually correct Ayurvedically that you might not be too thrilled about rolling out of bed early in the morning—especially in winter/spring, the Kapha time of year, when animals hibernate, it's dark in the morning, and everyone feels more like staying under the covers a while longer. But, also speaking from an Ayurvedic point of view, it's very important to get out of bed and get moving before *even more* sluggish Kapha energy can accumulate. The longer you stay in bed, the more "Kapha" builds up and the more lethargic you will feel. Not surprisingly, it's usually the Kaphas of the world who are least likely to "get going." Vatas, because they simply find it impossible to stop moving, and Pittas, because they are so goal oriented, are much more likely to have some kind of exercise program already incorporated into their life. In fact, most fitness professionals are either Pittas or Pitta/Vatas who need to beware *overtraining*. But for everyone, it's important to make exercise a priority—right up there with showering and brushing your teeth. If you do that, you'll be amazed how much more alert you'll begin to feel. I know there will be many mornings when you don't *want* to get moving, but those of us who do exercise know that we'll feel better afterward. We don't always want to, but we know it will help.

It's not my intention here to lay out any one specific exercise program. In fact, considering the differences among body and personality types, lifestyles, and needs, that would be a virtually impossible task. What I will do, however, is describe the various types of exercise—strength/resistance training, aerobics, and flexibility training—and indicate which kinds, in which combinations, would be best for each of the three body types, depending, of course, on individual goals.

VATA, PITTA, KAPHA—WHAT YOU ARE DETERMINES HOW YOU MOVE

Vatas, as I'm sure you know by now, simply can't sit still. If you're a Vata, you're probably doing more aerobics than is good for you— spinning, stepping, and running until you drop. In this chapter I'm going to tell you about ways to balance all those aerobic activities with some strength training to increase lean muscle, and yoga, tai chi, or Pilates to "ground" you and calm you down. While you probably don't need to lose any more body fat, you do need to build lean muscle, relieve some of your stress, and support your nervous system. But don't panic, my goal is to balance and nurture your tired, wired adrenal glands and nervous system, not make you sit still. On the contrary, I know perfectly well that imbalanced Vatas *can't* sit still.

Although you would benefit from quiet, peaceful meditation, seated meditation is especially challenging for an imbalanced Vata, and movement—doing something like yoga or tai chi—is imperative.

Pittas are most biologically adapted to develop muscle, but because they are so competitive, they are likely to push themselves beyond their capacity. They need to be aware that lifting and running until they develop high blood pressure or suffer a heart attack is not a healthy way to approach fitness. If you're a Pitta, you may be walking that treadmill at a slant resembling Mr. Everest or challenging Mr. America to a bench-pressing contest. For you, adding Pilates and a cooling, calming yoga class to your program may be the answer, because both are a little slower and more controlled than other types of exercise—two qualities you'd do well to try to develop. The goal is to harness all that amazing type A energy the way a martial arts master does, so that you become *more* efficient and productive with less stress and strain.

Kaphas are the most exercise resistant and, of course, the ones who would benefit most from getting themselves moving and cranking up their metabolism. If you're a Kapha, the very thought of cardiovascular exercise may be anathema to you, but once you get in the groove and discover a program you like—be it yoga, Pilates, weightlifting, or walking—you'll probably find that you're beginning to feeling lighter and less sluggish. Combining cardiovascular activity with strength training for increased lean muscle and yoga for increased strength and stimulation will provide a well-rounded program you can live with and enjoy.

STRENGTH/RESISTANCE TRAINING

Strength training, also called resistance training, is defined as the use of resistance to build maximum muscle force. The resistance can be supplied by weights; by isometric contractions, as in yoga; or by water, as in swimming.

Strength training is an essential component of any exercise program, no matter what your body type. Unfortunately, many women in particular are reluctant to start lifting weights because they're afraid of "bulking up." Instead they continue to eat a low-fat diet and do more and more aerobics, and they can't understand why they don't get the results they want; in fact, many increase their body fat and become even more frustrated. The fact is, done correctly, strength training with weights doesn't cause women to develop bulk; it can, however, create a longer, leaner body with good definition. And as Olympic strength-training coach Charles Poliquin has said over and over again, "If you want to stay fat, just eat bagels and do aerobics."

Now that you know enough about balancing good fats, clean proteins, and nonstarchy, nongluten carbohydrates to avoid blood sugar swings and curb your cravings, and you understand why the bagel diet is not a good idea, the additional piece of information that you—like so many other people—may not yet have understood is why aerobic exercise alone is not the best way to lose weight or body fat. Aerobic exercise is important, of course, for cardiovascular health, and we'll be talking about that as well, but it shouldn't be the *only* form of exercise for anyone.

Think of the average male marathon runner. He may be thin—even skinny—because he's utilized most of his body fat. He will also have a strong cardiovascular system, but he doesn't have much muscle definition or tone and is usually susceptible to injuries. I see this myself all the time among the endurance athletes living in Boulder. Many of them don't want to take the time for strength training, and as a consequence, they are constantly injuring their knees or hips or backs!

Increasing lean muscle is important if you are trying to lose body fat, prevent osteoporosis, or just look tighter, harder, and more defined. As an adjunct to weight loss, building lean muscle will speed up your metabolism so that you'll be burning more calories just by being alive! According to Dr. Mauro DiPasquale, author of *The Anabolic Diet* and one of the leading experts in obesity research, adding one pound of lean muscle will allow you to burn fifty additional calories a day. Adding four pounds of lean muscle could thus allow you to burn up to two hundred additional calories a day. Too many people still believe that if they just eat fewer calories and forget the exercise, they will lose weight. But they're wrong. Unfortunately, it simply doesn't work that way. On the contrary, it has been proved in studies over and over again that cutting back too severely on calories can actually cause the metabolism to slow down. If you remember what I said earlier about homeostasis, you'll see that we are genetically engineered to maintain the status quo. And if we don't eat enough, our bodies will determine that we are starving and will automatically try to conserve whatever calories we do take in. Think of this as the flip side of the American "more must be better" theory: if eating less increases weight loss, then eating even less than what's recommended will accelerate the process. Not so!

Stay Off the Scale!

Weighing in is another mistake made by many women who still can't seem to believe that starving in order to see that number going down on the scale simply doesn't work in the long run. They would be better off eating a healthy diet, including sufficient calories and good fats, and incorporating some strength training into their fitness routine to build lean muscle while decreasing their percentage of body fat. The scale means very little and it drives people crazy. Think about a professional football player. While he may be 6 feet tall and weigh in at 290 pounds (technically overweight or even obese), at 6 percent body fat he's a lean mean machine. You want to go by how you look in your bathing suit or naked in front of the mirror, *not* what the scale says. Look at any female athlete—you would usually be surprised to find out how much she "weighs" even though she's tight and well defined.

For Kaphas, whose digestion tends to be slow in any case, and for Pittas, who may gain weight more easily than they lose it, doing some strength training is essential for optimum metabolic efficiency. But it's also critical for Vatas, who most likely don't have a problem with weight management, but whose bones are usually small and more brittle than those of Pittas or Kaphas. For them, building lean muscle and bone density can mean the difference between good health and debilitating osteoporosis in later life. Remember that after age sixty we will all enter the Vata time of life, which means that thin, small Vatas need to be extremely conscientious about remaining strong *before* they get to that point.

Core Strength Training

Pilates, developed by physical trainer Joseph Pilates in the 1920s, is a form of resistance and flexibility training that is particularly important for building core strength. Your core is your body's center of power, and it is vital to strengthen the core muscles, such as those around the spinal cord and in the abdomen, to avoid injuries, particularly to the lower back, as well as to develop good posture and more efficient movement. If you want strong, flat abdominal muscles, check out Pilates!

No matter what your constitutional type, you will benefit from incorporating Pilates or some other form of core strengthening into your program because all of us need to develop well-balanced back and abdominal muscles to stand straight and tall, provide support for our skeletal structure, and prevent injury to the extremities, particularly when engaging in sports.

Doing a hundred crunches or situps to strengthen abdominal muscles is no longer considered productive in the fitness world because these are not movements we actually perform in the course of normal activity, and they can eventually shorten the abdominal muscles, leading to curvature of the spine and poor posture. People who sit at a desk or computer all day—as so many of us do—already have a tendency toward developing a forward head and curvature of the spine, so they need to strengthen and *stretch* (not shorten) their core abdominal muscles and spine. Paul Chek, owner of the C.H.E.K. Institute and a well-known corrective exercise specialist in the field of orthopedic rehabilitation who certifies personal trainers and medical fitness professionals, has said: "The body is designed to function in balance. There should be balance between the core abdominal muscles, neck, hips and hip flexors, and the extremities to create a strong, functionally fit body." Pilates, combined with strength training, can achieve this. In martial arts they refer to your core or center as your *hara*. It's your place of strength and balance. In yoga, steadiness and strength are also two of the most important teachings.

AEROBICS/CARDIOVASCULAR FITNESS

When we discuss fitness in general, we are usually referring to a person's aerobic capacity or cardiovascular endurance, which measures the degree of efficiency with which your heart and lungs are able to deliver oxygenated, nutrient-rich blood to the working muscles and organs and remove "spent" or "depleted" blood and metabolic waste products during physical exertion. In practical terms, this is a measure of "functional fitness," or your capacity to climb stairs, carry heavy packages, or run for the bus without huffing and puffing. In other words, the fitter you are, the less strain there will be on your cardiovascular system when you exert yourself. In a *New York Times* article of October 24, 2000, health expert Jane Brody writes that doing just twenty minutes of cardiovascular activity at a time, three times a week, can increase the benefits of any fitness program.

The goal is really just to do *something* to improve your cardiovascular health, even if it is only twice a week in the beginning. For Kaphas, who will benefit most from aerobic activity, even a brisk twenty-minute walk would be helpful. One of the more stimulating forms of yoga, such as Ashtanga, might be a good way to start. Pittas would do well with moderate levels of aerobic activity, such as taking a dance class, cross-country skiing, biking, or swimming. Because of their "hot" nature, they usually enjoy cooling outdoor exercise, but running at noon in July wouldn't be a good idea. As I've said before, Vatas really do need to move (and, of course, everyone needs the health benefit of some aerobic activity), but they don't need to be spinning any faster than they already are, so for you Vatas I'd suggest dancing, swimming, walking, and some light biking—all in moderation.

Interval Training

Even weight training, although it is generally considered to be an anaerobic exercise, can provide aerobic activity if you move through the program quickly, and particularly if you combine it with interval training. If you are already in relatively good physical shape and want to mobilize fat while still maintaining lean muscle, interval training can help. Remember what we said a few pages back about those skinny marathoners? If you compare their body composition with that of sprinters, you'll understand why moving very quickly for short periods of time can help you to maintain lean muscle while you also lose fat, so that you look stronger and harder. Depending on your level of fitness, long-duration, low-intensity cardiovascular exercise alone may not be the right way to achieve the results you are seeking. As it is in diet, variety is the key to a good exercise program.

Assuming you are relatively fit and in good health, you might want to try this. Following your strength workout, pedaling a bike or running as fast as you can in good form for twenty to forty seconds, then slowing it down for forty-five to sixty seconds, and then repeating these intervals for twenty to thirty minutes will increase your lactic acid levels, and to quote Olympic strength-training coach Charles Poliquin once again: "Since growth hormone levels rise as a function of increased lactic acid levels, this powerful anticatabolic hormone will help you to lose body fat while maintaining lean muscle." Finding a qualified fitness professional to help get you started might be a great idea. Coach Poliquin is known in the fitness industry for turning out lean, strong athletes safely and quickly. His German Body Composition Program is very effective for increasing muscle and decreasing body fat. Qualified trainers may be found on his web site (see page 313).

FLEXIBILITY/STRESS MANAGEMENT

Flexibility is determined by measuring your range of motion around a joint. Maintaining flexibility is, obviously, important for everyone, but it's particularly important as we age. My own parents live in Flushing, Queens, which has the second largest Korean population outside of Seoul, Korea. A wonderful man named Peter Wong, who is seventy-five years old, leads a group of people in Tai Chi in the local park almost every morning, rain or shine. The twenty to thirty participants range in age from forty to eighty-plus, and it is wonderful to watch them going through the slow, balletic movements in unison but at their own pace. One of the major challenges to functional fitness as we age is that we lose our ability to contract any given muscle in the body at any given time, which means that we lose our agility. But I've watched elderly Asians squatting comfortably in their yards or gardens, tending their flowers, and I've seen the same thing in Africa, Peru, Ecuador, or any place where life is more physically demanding than in our high-tech, motorized culture. It just proves to me that getting old does not mean that we have to become weak, frail, or brittle.

Tai Chi

Nikki Winston, who at the time we met was the Tai Chi instructor at the Golden Door Spa in Escondido, California, explains Tai Chi as a kind of "moving meditation" that draws upon nature in order to help people return balance and harmony to their day-to-day existence. Its movements are a reflection of the "dance" between nature and the elements—wind, water, fire, wood, and metal—and are intended to increase our connection to both.

Chi means "vital life force" or "energy" (comparable to *prana* in Ayurveda), and Tai Chi begins by helping participants to find their center, or core strength, which is where *chi* is stored. It can have a profound impact on the immune system (or *ojas* in Ayurveda) and on our ability to handle stress and tension by helping us to move more naturally and freely, and it can ultimately increase flexibility and balance, which is particularly important for older people, whose bones can become more brittle, exposing them to serious injury when they fall. As a discipline, it can help people to feel more grounded, centered, and relaxed, while improving awareness and alertness at the same time.

Yoga

While Tai Chi is one form of meditation and relaxing flexibility exercise, yoga is actually considered the sister science to Ayurveda. Traditionally, yoga was the means for achieving spiritual self-realization, while Ayurveda dealt with the physical and emotional aspects of life. Together, they strive to restore the wholeness of body, mind, and spirit.

While the more spiritual aspects of yoga practice have been largely de-emphasized in the United States, yoga actually consists of three basic components: the postures or poses, called asanas; breath work (or pranyama); and meditation. Asana actually means "right posture," and the asanas are intended to achieve a sustained and comfortable position that will allow you to engage in controlled deep breathing, which will in turn facilitate meditation.

The way you breathe can have a significant effect on both your nervous system and your digestive system. Certain kinds of breathing can help to heat you up or cool you down. If your breath is short and up in your throat and chest, you are in fight-or-flight mode, activating your sympathetic nervous system and telling your body that it is experiencing some kind of emergency. And, as we've discussed, living the stress-filled American life has made this a day-to-day experience for too many people. Simply becoming conscious of breathing deeply into your lower stomach, learning the deep yogic breathing techniques, can signal your body that it's okay to relax. Your parasympathetic nervous system is then stimulated, telling your body the emergency is over. That's one of the reasons Ayurveda suggests you relax quietly for a few minutes after lunch—your largest meal—so that your nervous system has a chance to calm down, allowing your digestive system to do its work. Try it for yourself and see what happens. After lunch, close your door or sit on a park bench or just lower the back of your car seat. Put your hands on your belly so that you can actually feel it rising and falling, and try to breathe deeply. Try saying a mantra like "Breath in" on your inhale and "Breathe out" on your exhale, or say "So" as you inhale and "Hum" as you exhale. You might even want to be like the Karate Kid and say "Wax on" for the inhale and "Wax off" for the exhale. Saying a mantra, which we have all come to associate with meditation, is actually the simple repetition of a phrase that is calming and focusing. It may take some practice, but after a while you'll actually feel your mind calming down and your focus returning.

Meditation has been described by writer Angela Hynes in *Shape* magazine as "deep physical relaxation combined with acute mental alertness," or, as it's expressed in *Nutrition in Complementary Care*, a publication of the American Dietetic Association, "no more and no less than being present in the moment." This can mean anything from sitting quietly, walking through the woods, gardening, dancing, doing Tai Chi or yoga, or even lifting weights with proper breathing and focused attention. One-pointed focus is a skill taught in both yoga and martial arts.

While any kind of exercise, if we are "present in the moment," can help us to relax and focus, the various yoga postures, or asanas, are designed specifically for that pupose. They can range from extremely gentle to rather strenuous, and different forms of yoga can be more or less beneficial for each of the constitutional types. Following are descriptions of the most common styles of yoga.

Hatha yoga and traditional Integral yoga are calm, slow-moving, gentle forms that encourage attention to proper alignment of your body and to the health of the inner organs. Through the postures of Hatha yoga we are able to maintain a balance of strength, flexibility, and relaxation, not only in the yoga class, but in our daily approach to life. This is excellent for Vatas and Pittas because these postures place a lot of emphasis on breathing and deep relaxation.

Ashtanga is yoga for those who want a more serious workout. It is physically demanding as participants move through a series of flows, jumping from one posture to another in order to build strength, flexibility, and stamina. There are various levels of difficulty. Vatas and Pittas might do well in level one, but levels two and three can be too stimulating. Ashtanga is a great form of exercise for Kaphas.

Bikrams is performed in an extremely hot room. Participants move through a series of twenty-six poses, repeated twice, and should be prepared to sweat. This form of yoga is designed to warm and stretch the muscles, ligaments, and tendons in a particular order. Vatas and Kaphas usually love Bikrams, but it's often too heating for Pittas. It is good, however, for helping type A personalities learn how to go into relaxation quickly, because it requires that you hold a pose and then relax over and over again.

Iyengar yoga involves a series of standing postures performed while paying great attention to the precise alignment of your body. It is known not only for its attention to details, but also for its use of props such as blocks and belts. This form can be helpful for all three constitutional types.

There are several other types of yoga, including Anusara, Kundalini, Svaroopa, and Viniyoga, that we'll not be discussing here, but if you are interested in finding out more about them, I've listed some excellent sources (see page 309).

As a form of exercise, yoga can increase both flexibility and strength, but perhaps its most important benefit is to help reduce stress. In its original and purest form, yoga is, in fact, a kind of meditation. According to Stephen Cope, author of *Yoga and the Quest for the True Self,* "Many important yogic scriptures say that hatha yoga should be practiced in the context of raja yoga (the yoga of meditation)," and meditation, as we've just discussed, can have a powerful stress-reducing effect. I've been saying all along that by balancing your stress, you will be less inclined to turn to food as a counterproductive stress management technique, and I have experienced firsthand how little I need to eat after just an hour of meditation and yoga. My mind and nervous system are so calm that food isn't really in my thoughts.

Many of you—especially type A Pittas and spinning Vatas—may not have thought of yoga as "real" exercise, or maybe you tried it and didn't like it. But as I know from my own experience, and from having seen and worked with so many "Vata'd out" fitness fanatics, you are the ones who would really benefit from a day of relaxing, rejuvenating yoga rather than another killer workout. Perhaps you tried a type of yoga or took a class at a time of day that wasn't suited to your constitutional type, or maybe you simply haven't found the right teacher for you. Yoga can be beneficial for everyone, and therapeutic yoga can enhance virtually any weight management program. I can't urge you too strongly to try it again! Many people think yoga is all about getting into pretzel positions that are impossible for a mortal individual, but that is not yoga. Therapeutic yoga can help anyone from an obese, sedentary person to a person with cancer, to an elite athlete. The benefits of combining breath, awareness, and movement are very powerful. The asanas should be done with "steadiness and sweetness." They should feel good and not cause pain. Otherwise it's not yoga.

Here are some suggestions for the types of yoga and for particular poses that would be best for Vatas, Pittas, and Kaphas. You can do these anywhere—at home, in a hotel room, even in your office when you're feeling out of balance.

Yoga for Vatas

On an emotional level, for Vatas or those in a Vata imbalance, a gentle Hatha yoga class with slow, nurturing, supportive postures will create peace, calm, and balance. On a physical level, there are many breathing techniques and yoga postures that will help to alleviate the Vata tendency toward bloating, constipation, and gas and keep the digestive system working more efficiently. Because Vatas have so much of the air element in their systems, seated poses that are closer to the ground can be very helpful.

Many fitness professionals are overtraining and in a Vata imbalance. In addition, anyone who travels frequently, especially on a frenetic business schedule, is likely to be in a Vata imbalance and suffering from jet lag, insomnia, anxiety, and overstimulation. But whatever its cause, an excess of Vata can be calmed and brought back into balance with a few simple yoga exercises. Remember that whatever your constitutional type, you need to pay attention to the imbalance you're in at the moment.

The best Vata-pacifying yoga poses put emphasis on the pelvic region and colon (which are the main Vata sites) and help to calm the nervous system, keep you grounded, and aid digestion. Here are a few you might want to try, especially if you're in a Vata imbalance: Don't forget to take a few deep belly breaths as you move into and out of the postures and always start with a slight pelvic tilt in all exercises. In lying-down postures, simply tilt your pelvis up to the ceiling so your lower back straightens and gently touches the floor. In standing postures, make sure your feet are hip-distance apart, knees slightly bent, and pelvis gently tucked under (do not arch your back). Do that a few times with the breath to get familiar with it.

The Knee to Chest Pose (or the Wind-Releasing Pose) can actually help to alleviate gas, bloating, and constipation.

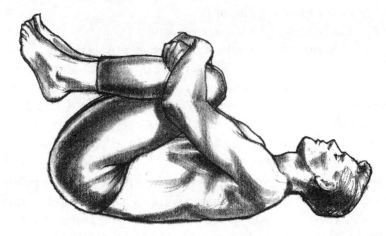

Lie on your back with your legs and arms straight along the floor in a comfortable position. Bend your knees so that the soles of your feet are flat on the floor and tilt your pelvis slightly to the ceiling so your lower back is on the floor; you should *not* feel much space between your back and the floor. Hold there for one or two deep breaths and release. Lift your feet off the floor and bring your knees toward your chest. Take hold of your knees (do not cause unnecessary pressure on your knees; if you have bad knees take hold of the backs of your thighs just below your knees) and take a few deep breaths.

If you want to go further with this pose, straighten your right leg, keeping it off the floor, while your left knee remains close to your chest. Bring your right knee back to your chest and straighten your left leg. Repeat these movements several times.

When done, hug both knees into your chest with your hands under your knees. If you like, you can rock from side to side, holding your legs to relax your back.

To come out of the pose, release your legs and bring the soles of your feet back to the floor with your knees still bent. Then straighten your arms and legs along the floor and relax with a few deep belly breaths before standing up.

Seated Forward Bends can calm and ground you when you are feeling spacey and overwhelmed. See Pitta poses below.

Child's Pose can help to ground, soothe, and nurture a stressed-out system.

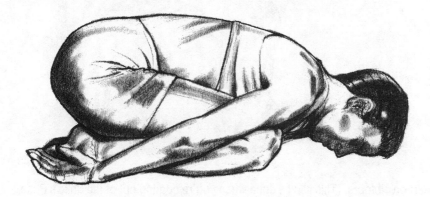

Start on your hands and knees with your hands below your shoulders and your knees below your hips.

Widen your knees slightly and tilt your pelvis just a drop forward to straighten your lower back.

Slowly lower your hips toward your heels and bring your upper body and head down toward the floor.

If it's hard to bring your hips to your heels, widen your knees more or place a pillow or blanket between your hips and your heels by positioning it on top of your legs, under your butt.

You have a few choices for different hand positions:

To get a good extension and to stretch your back, stretch your arms out on the floor in front of you. You can also slightly walk your fingertips away from you to lengthen the stretch.

For relaxation, you can either make a pillow with your hands and rest your head on your hands, or you can rest your arms on the floor at your sides with your hands reaching back toward your heels.

Breathe deeply and relax.

To come out of the pose, place the palms of your hands on the floor and press into the floor. Slowly bring your hips off your heels and come back onto all fours.

Cat Pose is good for mobility and flexibility of the spine.

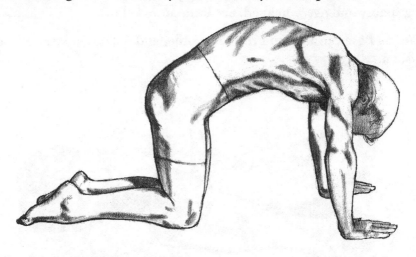

Start on all fours. (This can be done when you're coming out of the Child's Pose.)

As you inhale, gently arch your back up so that you look like a Halloween cat. Move and roll your whole spine into a slight arch, so that you are not scrunching just your shoulders. If this is uncomfortable for your back, keep it straight or in a neutral position and gently tuck your pelvis under a little bit.

As you exhale, move from the bottom of your spine, bring the tip of your spine up, as a cat does when trying to stick out its tail. After your tailbone tilts up, arch the rest of your back down, moving your spine fluidly in a downward direction.

Then, as you inhale again, slowly arch your back up. As you do the pose, feel the stretch and elongation in your spine. Feel how your spine is releasing any tension you are holding in your back.

Repeat several cycles of this movement.

After several cycles, return to a neutral stance on your hands and knees.

You can then roll onto your back to do a Lying Down Spinal Twist.

Lying Down Spinal Twist can improve digestion and reduce the feeling of "spaciness" that is a problem for Vatas when they become overwhelmed.

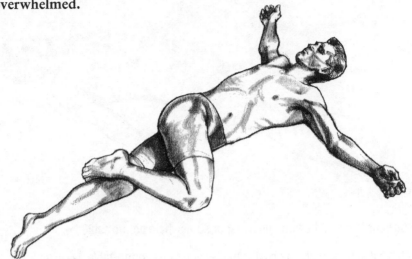

Lie flat on your back on the floor with your legs extended straight out.

Bring your arms away from your body on the floor until they are extended straight out from your shoulders in a "T" formation.

Bend one knee and place the sole of that foot on the floor.

Press the sole of your foot into the floor, lift your hips, and move them slightly to one side, in the same direction as your bent knee so that your leg is lined up with your neck and head; you should be one long line.

Lift the foot that is on the floor and bring it to rest gently on top of your straight leg.

Drop your knee over your straight leg toward the floor.

Turn your head in the opposite direction your bent knee is moving.

Your knee doesn't have to come all the way to the floor and your shoulder doesn't have to stay on the floor. You can put a pillow under your knee if there is too much strain on your back. Breathe deeply.

To come out of the pose, lift your knee up toward the ceiling and bring the sole of your foot back to the floor.

Bring your hips back to center.

Repeat on the other side.

Relaxation Pose is one of the most important in any yoga routine.

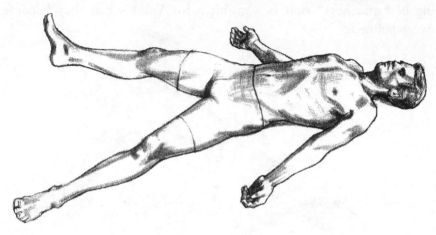

Lie on your back on the floor, on a mat or somewhere comfortable.

Stretch out and, depending on what makes you most comfortable, leave your hands straight along your sides or let them rest lightly on your body. Leave your legs straight on the floor or, if your lower back is not comfortable, bend your knees slightly or put a pillow or blanket under your knees or your ankles.

As you rest in this pose, bring your attention to following your breath. Feel yourself relax deeply with each inhalation, and with each exhalation, feel yourself let go of any tension or stress in your body. Keep your eyes closed so you are not becoming distanced but are allowing your attention to focus on a growing sensation of calm and quiet.

Stay in the pose as long as you feel comfortable, at least 5 to 10 minutes. It may be hard to relax without falling asleep, but deep rest other than sleep is very important to health.

To come out of the pose, roll onto your side and come to sitting from this position. Rolling onto your side before sitting up puts less stress on your lower back.

Other poses that might be helpful for calming Vata are Sun Salutation, Tree Pose, Extended Triangle, Revolving Triangle, Forward Bends, and Cobra. It would be best to ask a qualified yoga instructor about them. A yoga instructor who has some knowledge of Ayurveda would be ideal. See the resource section.

Yoga for Pittas

For the overheated Pitta, who is cranky and irritable because he or she has been doing too much, there are poses that put pressure on the liver and gallbladder and help to reduce excess heat and irritability. Until I understood this, I used to laugh when my yoga instructor said a certain pose was working on the liver or the colon, but now I understand that moving in particular ways will create specific responses in your body. Much more than simply building muscle or increasing cardiovascular strength, these movements aid digestion and create emotional balance.

Because Pittas can be so competitive, they tend to be drawn to the more aggressive forms of yoga when they would really be best served by doing something gentle, calm, and soothing at least one day a week. Ashtanga yoga, for example, is more heating and athletic, and while it might be perfect for Kaphas who need to lose weight, it can be too stimulating, aggravating, and warming for the type A Pitta. Hatha or traditional Integral yoga would be very beneficial for a type A Pitta. At the end of one of these classes, Pittas should feel focused and slightly energized all day, but not overstimulated or cranky. And as I've already mentioned, the overheated Pitta should stay far away from the overheated Bikrams yoga classroom.

The following five postures will help to cool, relax, and soothe even the angriest Pitta:

Lying Down Spinal Twist. See Vata poses (page 121).

Seated Forward Bend

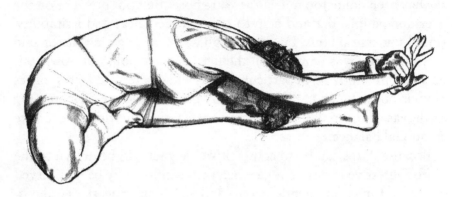

Sit on the floor with your legs straight out in front of you.

Bend one knee and place the sole of your foot on the floor.

Drop that knee to the side with the sole of your foot facing your straight leg.

Sit up with your back tall and extended and your pelvis slightly tilted under, not arched.

Fold forward from your hip joint over your straight leg, gently stretching the back of your leg, your hamstring, and your back. Go only as far as you can with a straight lower back for the first few breaths. Feel your body releasing.

Let your upper body relax, let your shoulders, neck, and head relax.

Place your hands on either side of your stretched leg, as far down the leg as is comfortable for you. If you feel tight while doing this, you can either bend your knee or place a small pillow or blanket under your knee.

Breathe deeply and relax.

To come out of the pose, gently roll your spine up, first the lower spine, then the middle spine, then the upper spine, until you are sitting up.

Unbend your bent knee and straighten your leg along the floor. Shake out both legs.

Repeat on the other side.

Triangle Pose **is energizing and strengthening, especially for the back.**

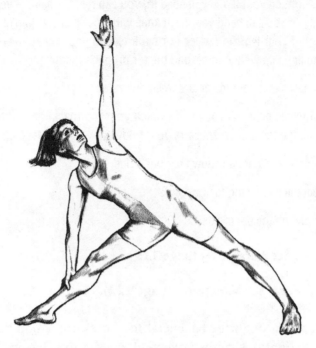

It's best to do this, or any standing pose, in bare feet, so that you don't slip on the floor. A yoga mat is highly recommended.

Stand with your feet about one leg's distance apart and facing forward.

Turn one foot out 90 degrees so it is facing away from your body (this will be your front foot).

Rise up on the toes of your other foot (the back foot) and gently slide your heel slightly out to the side.

Stop for a moment and get your balance, standing tall and extended with your pelvis slightly tucked under; do not arch your lower back.

On a deep inhalation, raise both arms to shoulder height with your fingertips reaching and extending out to either side.

Bend from your hips, reaching over your front leg and extending your front hand down toward your leg. At the same time, reach your back hand up toward the ceiling. Extend and reach through the fingertips of both hands.

Gently pull in your abdominal muscles by bringing your belly button in and up. Use your abdominal muscles to stabilize and support your back.

If you can, let your front hand rest, palm facing forward, in front of your leg without putting weight on your leg. If you need to, you can rest the palm of your hand on your thigh, or you can bend your front knee with your palm resting on your thigh or in front of your leg. Do not lock or hyperextend your knees; keep your knee "soft" and lined up with your second toe for proper alignment.

Take deep breaths into your lower abdomen and relax.

To come out of the pose, as you inhale, reach your top (back) hand up and out to the side, letting the movement carry your body back up to a standing position.

Gently let your arms float back down to your sides.

Turn both feet back to facing forward.

Repeat the pose on the other side.

Child's Pose. See Vata poses (page 119).

Relaxation Pose. See Vata poses (page 122).

Other poses that might be beneficial for Pittas are Moon Salutation, Slow Sun Salutations with movement on the exhalation, Shoulder Stand, Plow, Fish, Locust, Boat, Bridge, Camel, and Bow. Ask a qualified yoga instructor about them.

Yoga for Kaphas

Kaphas not only dislike moving more than is absolutely necessary, but because of their larger body type, they may also feel self-conscious in any kind of exercise class. Nevertheless, yoga is one form of exercise that can be extremely beneficial to the sluggish Kapha by stimulating the metabolism to burn body fat and opening up the chest area to relieve the Kapha tendency toward congestion. Beginners would do well to start with level one Ashtanga classes but can move on to level two, which, as I've mentioned, are fairly stimulating and keep the body moving. Bikrams yoga classes, which are held in a room that is usually heated to 95 degrees, can be as beneficially cleansing for the clogged-up Kapha.

Following are some of the postures most likely to stimulate the sluggish Kapha.

Seated Twist stimulates digestion and helps to gently stretch and relieve tension in the back.

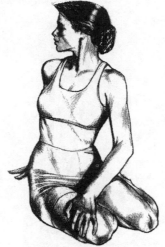

Kneel with your upper body straight upright and bring your hips to the floor to the right side of your legs so that you are sitting with your legs bent to your left. Or, you can start by sitting with your knees bent and your feet on the floor. Pick your feet up one at a time and place your legs to your left side.

Place your left hand on your right leg, above the knee. As you inhale, feel yourself becoming taller and try to straighten your lower back, but don't arch.

As you exhale, bring your right hand to rest on the floor to the side of, and slightly behind, your body so that you are gently twisting your lower back to the degree that is comfortable for you.

Keep your neck in line with your body; do not turn it to look behind you. You want your back to twist, not your neck.

As you remain in the twist for several breaths, feel yourself becoming taller with each inhalation and feel yourself relax more deeply into the twist with each exhalation.

To come out of the pose, bring your right hand off the floor and come back to center.

Switch the position of your feet to the right side, put your right hand on your left leg, above the knee, and bring your left hand to the side of, and slightly behind your body.

Complete the twist to the left side.

Standing Chest Opener is great for helping you to breathe more deeply, feel more energized, and reduce the tension in your shoulders.

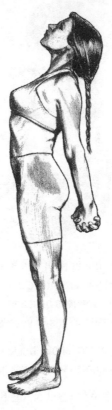

In your bare feet to maximize balance, stand comfortably with your weight equally distributed over both feet, your knees slightly bent, and your pelvis slightly tucked forward. This is a posture in itself: Mountain Pose, or Tadasasana, is one of the most important for proper posture and alignment for all other postures. Look in the mirror and notice if your head sticks out or your back is curved.

Standing straight, let your shoulders roll up and back and down.

Reach both arms behind you, clasp the fingers of both hands behind your back, and gently stretch by lifting your hands up behind you as far as is comfortable while you arch your chest forward.

To come out of the pose, bring your hands back down, relax your chest, unclasp your fingers, and bring your arms back down to your sides. You can shake your arms and roll your shoulders up and back and down again.

Repeat the pose several times.

Warrior Pose

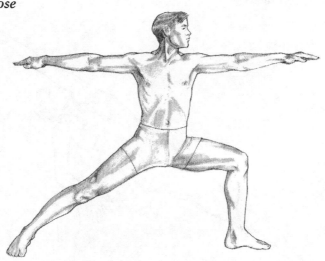

In your bare feet, stand with your legs about one leg's length apart and one foot turned at a 90-degree angle so that it is facing away from your body (this will be your front foot).

Rise up on the toes of your other (back) foot and gently drop your heel to the outside so that your front heel is aligned with the arch of your back foot. Keep your body facing center, even though you may want to turn toward your front foot.

Bring your arms up and out to your sides at shoulder height, extending through your fingertips and keeping your shoulders relaxed.

Bend your front knee so that it is behind your ankle. If your knee is in front of your ankle when you bend your leg, you need a wider stance. Putting your knee in front of the ankle will strain the knee joint. Make sure your knee is lined up with the center of your heel, and your pelvis is tucked under. Try not to arch your lower back.

You can look over your front hand if that is comfortable for your neck, or you can continue to face forward.

Remain in the pose for a few to several breaths, as long as feels comfortable without straining. While in the pose, keep your shoulders, neck, and jaw relaxed. Keep reaching your fingertips out as if you had wings and keep your front knee bent. This pose is very strengthening.

From the Warrior Pose, move into the Side Stretch Pose, which follows.

Side Stretch Pose

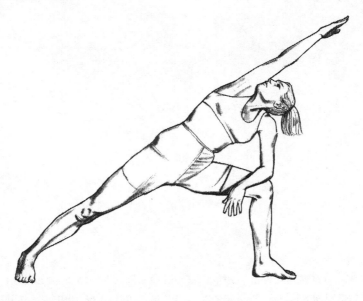

Keep your front knee bent (as in the Warrior Pose), bend the elbow of your front arm down toward your body, and rest your forearm on your thigh. Make sure again that your knee is not passing your ankle. Your lower leg should be perpendicular to the floor.

Sweep your back arm up above your head, and reach your hand over your head and in front of you. Look up toward this side of your body.

Feel your whole body stretching from your fingertips down your side and down your back leg. Make sure you are not arching your lower back.

Breathe and stretch.

To come out of the pose, reach up with your top (back) hand and let your hand carry your body back to center.

Let your hands come back down to your sides and straighten your front leg.

Turn both feet so that they are facing forward.

Repeat the Warrior Pose and the Side Stretch to the other side.

Abdominal Roll with Bent Knees is useful for improving digestion, weight loss, reducing lower back pain, and strengthening the abdominal muscles.

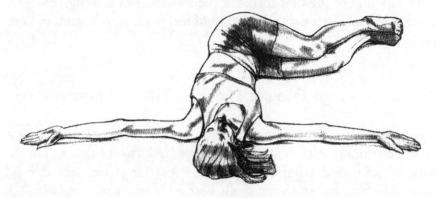

Lie on your back with your knees bent, the soles of your feet on the floor, and your pelvis slightly tucked.

Bring your arms out from your shoulders to form a "T."

Lift your feet off the floor and drop both knees to your right side as you inhale. Your back will twist gently and your left shoulder may come off the floor. You can bring your knees toward the floor, but they don't have to move all the way to the floor.

As you exhale, bring both knees up off the floor and over the center of your body with your feet on the floor.

As you inhale, drop both knees to the left side. On the exhale, bring both knees back to center. It's important that you do this movement on the exhale since this is when you are exerting yourself and using your abdominal muscles.

Repeat to both sides as many times as is comfortable for you, slowly increasing the number of repetitions on each side.

When you're finished, let your legs stretch out on the floor, place your hands wherever is comfortable, and spend a few minutes relaxing and focusing on your breathing.

Some additional poses that might be beneficial to Kapha are Sun Salutation, Shoulder Stand, Lion, Plow, Fish, Downward Dog, and Back Bend. Ask a qualified yoga instructor about these. An overweight person may need some modifications to the traditional postures at the beginning. Therapeutic yoga can be done with a chair and modified for people with weight problems, injuries, cancer, diabetes, or other problematic conditions. Don't think you can't do it—it's really one of the best forms of mental and physical movement if done safely and properly, and it should feel good so you want to keep going!

DETERMINING THE EXERCISE PROGRAM THAT IS RIGHT FOR YOU

You now know that it's important to combine strength and cardiovascular training with flexibility and stress reduction exercise, but the proper ratios and combinations, like everything else, will depend upon who you are and what goals you want to set for yourself. Ask yourself the following questions:

> What is my body type?
> What is my personality type?
> What are my goals?
> What imbalances am I experiencing?

By now you've already determined your personality and body type, and you know whether your goal is to be a competitive bodybuilder; to lose fifty pounds; to look harder, leaner, and tighter; or simply to avoid injuries and osteoporosis later in life. But the last question still remains the big one. Remember our earlier discussion of adrenal exhaustion? If you're a type A Pitta who's always trying to do another ten reps, or if you've been pushing too hard for too long and find that you need three cups of coffee or two Diet Cokes to get going in the morning or through the afternoon, chances are that your adrenal glands are exhausted. If that's the case, forcing yourself through another spinning class or running extra miles isn't going to help. A soothing, calming, rejuvenating yoga class, on the other hand, may be just what you need. It's true that energy creates energy, so exercise is *always* important, but the *kind* of exercise you need may change with your circumstances.

The goal of Ayurveda is to teach you how to listen to your body so that you learn not only when you need to move, but also when you need to stop. As I told you in the introduction, I had to learn this the hard way by tearing the ligament in my knee. But now I understand that if I wake up feeling really tired, rather than pushing myself through a weight-training workout, I'm better off going to a gentle yoga class to cool, calm, and ground myself. Then, if I get a good night's sleep, my weight workout is invariably more productive the next day.

BEFORE YOU BEGIN

There are certain "rules" everyone should learn to follow before starting to exercise in order to get the most out of their program and, above all, prevent injury.

- Always warm up by doing at least 5 minutes of walking or light biking or lifting to get the blood flowing to your muscles.
- Never weight-train directly after a yoga class. Lifting weights after static stretching is contraindicated: muscles are temporarily weakened after static stretching owing to the relaxation response, and are therefore more likely to pull or tear or be injured. Yoga after weight training would be fine.
- Always pay attention to your breathing. You should try to keep your breath deep in your lower abdomen. Shallow breathing is an indication that your body is in fight-or-flight mode (in other words, under stress), and *holding* your breath can increase your blood pressure. Breathing *in* through your nose and *out* through your nose is very balancing and actually puts you in a more meditative place with less oxidative stress on the body. This is very important for athletes because, again, too much of a good thing is not a good thing! Excessive exercise in bad form causes oxidative breakdown and injuries.
- Before starting a new fitness program, it would be best to consult with your physician as well as a qualified fitness professional in your area. Please see our resource section for suggestions.

SUGGESTED EXERCISE PROGRAMS FOR
VATAS, PITTAS, AND KAPHAS

Without being too rigidly prescriptive, and assuming that you, as an individual, don't have any specific health problems that would require a specialized fitness program, here are some suggestions for a mix of strength, aerobic, flexibility, and stress-reducing exercises that would be appropriate for each of the three constitutional types. (If you do have a specific health problem, the National Fitness Therapy Association [see page 313] can help you find a medical fitness professional who is trained to work with that problem.

Obviously anyone training for a specific sport or event like bodybuilding or ultraendurance events would modify his or her program accordingly, but do make sure to keep core strength in mind.

Vatas

Strength/resistance training 2 to 3 times per week.

Hatha yoga or Tai Chi once or twice a week.

Cardiovascular or aerobic work no more than 20 to 30 minutes long (such as a nice brisk walk to yoga class), no more than 2 or 3 times a week, possibly after a weight workout. (I know you just laughed at that one!)

Try Interval training—good for working off excess energy while building lean muscle and increasing bone density.

Pilates, for variety and to increase core strength.

Pittas

Weight/strength/resistance training twice a week.

Hatha or Integral yoga, once or twice a week on a day when you do no other form of exercise.

Pilates twice a week (followed, if you like, by 20 to 30 minutes of interval training and a few yoga postures to cool down).

Recreational aerobic exercise such as biking, hiking, skiing, or swimming, on weekends and during leisure time.

Kaphas

Weight training with interval training 2 to 4 times a week.

Bikrams, Ashtanga, or another of the more aggressive forms of yoga twice a week, modified to the ability of the person.

Recreational aerobic activities such as running, hiking, or rowing on weekends.

Pilates is always beneficial for core strength—try 1 or 2 times a week.

Kaphas also have the hardest time getting motivated, so simply getting out of bed and walking for 10 to 30 minutes first thing in the morning would help get a sluggish system moving. Just do something; start small and try to be consistent.

THE BOTTOM LINE

Some kind of exercise program should be an essential part of everybody's fitness regimen, whatever his or her constitutional type. And that program should ideally involve a variety of activities including strength/resistance training, aerobic exercise, and flexibility training. But just as there is no one diet that will be appropriate for all people in all circumstances, so there is no one exercise program that will provide equal benefit for all.

Not only will the kinds of activities I've suggested in this chapter help you, whatever your constitutional type, to become physically fitter, leaner, and more toned, they will also, ultimately, help to calm and soothe whatever emotional imbalance you may be experiencing and to curb your cravings for sugary, oily, calming—but decidedly unhealthy—foods.

Exercise has been shown to increase the levels of endorphins and serotonin in the brain, making people feel better about themselves, while lack of exercise is equally shown to increase susceptibility to depression. The stress-reducing qualities of various physical activities have been well documented. Richard Ferguson, writing in *Running Journal,* has this to say about the reasons for experiencing a "runner's high": "Stress is a result of our perceptions of stressors [that result] in a hormonal response in the body that prepares us for physical action. In today's world we can't often act physically when stressed, like when the boss yells at us or we can't get a computer program to work right. Running can actually use up the stress hormones for their intended purpose, that being to prepare us for physical action!"

And it has equally been shown that relaxation techniques such as yoga and meditation have a beneficial effect on both mind and body. In Ayurveda, as I indicated earlier, yoga and meditation are virtually synonymous; as Alan Reder points out in the *Yoga Journal,* "Research indicates that meditation lowers bodily stress—which can lower blood pressure—reduces the risk of heart attacks and stroke by improving arterial health, and brings relief to chronic pain sufferers. Meditation has proven highly effective in treating psychological conditions, such as obsessive-compulsive disorder, depression, and anxiety." Meditation and yoga are also two of the key components of Dr. Dean Ornish's success in reversing heart disease without medication.

But to receive the full benefit of the stress-reducing effects of any exercise program, it is first necessary to be focused and present in the moment. This is, in fact, one of the areas in which yoga practitioners and sports fitness trainers are in total agreement. Reading or watching television while you pedal a stationary bike or use a treadmill is *not* being present in the moment, and I would suggest that if you dislike your current fitness program so much that you require these kinds of distractions, it is probably not the right program for you.

I hope there are enough alternatives offered in this chapter for you to discover the combination of activities that will both make you feel good and produce the most beneficial results.

CHAPTER SEVEN

Pulling It All Together

I realize that by this point you've received an enormous amount of information, and despite the fact that I've tried to keep reminding you of how all the pieces fit together, you may be feeling a bit overwhelmed. So I'd like to pause here and help you to assimilate everything you've learned—about Ayurveda; about how your body metabolizes proteins, fats, and carbohydrates; and about your food sensitivities—so that you can make it practical and applicable to your everyday life. As I've been saying all along, it should not be difficult, it should be pleasurable, but it is going to require that you pay attention—possibly more attention than you have in the past—to the signals your body is trying to send.

THE BASICS

First of all, as we've learned from Western nutritional science, it's important that we eat *something* at least every three hours. This is particularly important in our busy, overstressed society. If we were living in an ashram, or under very little stress, two meals a day might be plenty. In our modern, fast-paced world, however, most of us have overworked, depleted adrenal and hormonal systems and less than optimal digestion, and we need to fuel our bodies every three hours with some protein to prevent ourselves from "running on empty" and causing sugar and carbohydrate cravings. Eating more frequently than every three hours is not recommended in Ayurveda because we won't have properly digested our previous meal.

In addition to sufficient protein, we must also include sufficient *good oils* and *essential fatty acids* to maintain cellular integrity as well as to liquefy and mobilize plaque. Except for the lucky ones who have no problem digesting gluten, we should try to *decrease* the amount of *wheat- and gluten-based carbohydrates* in our diet, or at least to rotate them with nongluten grains, in order to minimize the risk of exacerbating the digestive problems that can result from overconsuming foods to which we are sensitive. And we should *increase* our consumption of nutrient-rich, *leafy green vegetables,* which will help to increase digestive efficiency. Above all, we should add as much *variety* as possible to our diet, not only to avoid increasing food sensitivities, but also to maximize the pleasure we derive from eating and keep our taste buds stimulated. And we should learn to *flavor our food with herbs and spices* so that it will be tastier and will satisfy our cravings, particularly for the sweet and soothing foods we seek in times of stress. So, to reiterate:

- Eat something every three hours.
- Include some protein in every meal.
- Be sure you are consuming enough good oils and essential fatty acids.
- Avoid overconsuming wheat- and gluten-based and/or starchy carbohydrates if you are gluten-sensitive and/or more prone to abdominal obesity.
- Increase your consumption of leafy green vegetables and cook them in a way that is appropriate for your constitutional type.
- Curb your cravings and increase your enjoyment by flavoring your food with herbs and spices.

It's been gratifying to me that the terms *balance, variety, digestion, taste,* and *satisfaction* can be heard more and more often these days both among hard-core bodybuilders and from members of the American Dietetic Association. It seems that East and West are at last coming together!

THE AYURVEDIC APPROACH

Ayurveda believes that to manage weight and achieve optimal health, we should be eating our main meal in the middle of the day, when digestion is strongest. (Remember that ten to two o'clock is the time of day associated with the Pitta constitutional type and that Pittas have the strongest digestion and appetite.) The exception to this rule would be for those who are truly "night people." If you are one—and you'll know if you are—you'll be eating your main meal a bit later, when your digestion is stronger. After eating, we should "walk one thousand steps," or for about five minutes, and then rest for five to ten minutes, preferably on the left side because it helps digestion by increasing the digestive fire. (Interestingly, most pregnant women seem to be more comfortable lying on their left side once they "start to show.")

We should then have another warm protein snack or meal between three and four o'clock to preempt the low-blood-sugar craving for coffee and sweets, then have a lighter dinner between six and eight o'clock—the Kapha time of day, when digestion is not as strong as it is at midday. By this time most of us have already become sluggish and sleepy, and Ayurveda suggests that we try to get to bed by ten o'clock. Then, when our Pitta kicks in again (between ten P.M. and two A.M.), our liver (the organ that governs Pitta) will be able to do its primary job of cleansing the system while we sleep (remember the analogy I gave you earlier about emptying the office trash), instead of having to work on digesting a heavy evening meal. Making your body process a heavy meal at the same time it is trying to cleanse is extremely inefficient and will lead to less than optimal digestion and, ultimately, weight gain. (This is another point on which Ayurveda and bodybuilders agree. Both tell us to eat 70 percent of our daily calories before seven P.M. and if we need an evening snack, to keep it light.) If you think you need an evening snack, it could be a light protein such as cottage or feta cheese and rice crackers or warm milk with protein and spices like cardamom or cinnamon to help you sleep.

Unfortunately, this is exactly the opposite of what most Americans do. Either because we're "too busy to eat" or because we think that if we starve ourselves (or save up our calories) all day we can indulge ourselves later, we literally run on empty between ten and two o'clock, the busiest, most stressful part of the day (and the time when we need the most fuel). Then we make up for it with a heavy, three-course meal between six and ten, just the Kapha time when we will have the most difficulty processing all that food. We don't include enough protein in our diet, we deprive ourselves of the good fats that will help us to "liquefy" and mobilize body fat, and we overload on the kinds of starchy, gluten-based carbohydrates that may trigger our food sensitivities and cause the blood sugar swings that lead to un-controllable cravings.

A Balanced Approach to the Perfect Ayurvedic Day

Based on what Ayurveda tells us about digestion, a perfect day would run something like this:*

- Wake up at sunrise, the Kapha time of day. The longer you stay in bed, the more lethargic you will feel.
- Meditate. Or, sit quietly and ask for what you'd like this day to bring. Give thanks if you'd like.
- Take your L-glutamine supplement, as suggested in chapter 9. Wait 10 minutes and have something light, such as ½ a piece of fruit, or some cottage cheese, or tea or a protein shake (pages 144, 146), if you feel you need to eat before exercising to get your blood sugar up. Everyone is different; some people need to eat a little light protein before they exercise. In general, how-ever, if you are trying to lose weight and/or heal digestion, it is most beneficial to take some L-glutamine, wait 10 minutes, and then eat ½ a piece of fruit.
- Exercise.
- Right after your workout, have a postworkout protein shake (pages 144, 146) to provide amino acids, glucose, and simple carbohydrates. This is another point on which Ayurveda and sports nutrition agree—after a workout, you need some simple carbohydrates to help drive the amino acids into your cells, be-cause sugar is a carrier of amino acids. Ayurveda uses honey as a

carrier for herbs because it helps to move the herbs into the tissues.

- Between seven and ten o'clock have a light to medium protein meal and some essential fatty acids, in the form of either flaxseed or fish oil.
- Eat your main meal between ten and two o'clock. (If you're in a job where these are your busiest hours, eat at eleven o'clock; don't wait until three.) This should include something warm, like soup, to start with (unless it's midsummer or you live in south Florida); lots of vegetables with some good oil, such as canola, ghee, olive, hemp, or sesame, and nice spices and flavorings; some protein, such as eggs, cottage cheese, or organic meat, fish, or poultry; a small amount of nongluten grain; and something sweet to finish the meal. Don't forget to take 2 EPA/DHA supplements or flaxseed oil capsules.
- Walk your "thousand steps," or for about 5 minutes. This could mean a walk around the block.
- Rest for 5 minutes, preferably on your left side. Or sit quietly on a bench or in your car, or simply close your office door to allow your nervous system a few minutes to concentrate on digestion.
- Make sure to have another meal that includes some protein between three and four o'clock.
- Finish your day with a light dinner between six and eight o'clock. Maybe even take a stroll after dinner—very European—to help your digestion.

That's the general outline, and if we all ate this way in America, we would be more in tune with our bodies' natural biological rhythms. We would be allowing our digestive system to work at its optimum level, we would be consuming the right macronutrients at the most efficient times, and we would ensure that, mentally and physically, we were providing ourselves with sufficient, good-quality fuel to accomplish and accommodate whatever life threw our way. I can't emphasize enough that the connection between the nervous system and the digestive system is extremely important. If you skip lunch, you will certainly be in a Vata imbalance by three P.M. and will be having *more cravings* for sugar and caffeine, exactly what your tired, stressed, adrenally overloaded body *doesn't* need, and you'll find yourself overeating when you get home.

*According to Sarasvati Buhrman, Ph.D.: Approximately 75 percent of North Americans are bimodal, or day people. About 20 percent are night people, and 5 percent fit into neither category. Based on this theory, a night person or one who needs to be at work too early to work out in the morning should try to get up by six A.M., do a small meditation or thank-you for the day, take your glutamine, and go out for a short walk—even if it's just around the block—to get the Kapha moving and wake you up a bit.

Then have a light to medium breakfast, depending on your appetite, take your EFAs or flaxseed oil, and go to work. Have a small protein snack about three hours later to keep your blood sugar steady until lunch.

Eat a larger lunch, walk, and rest. If you start everything later because you are a night person, pay attention to when you are most hungry—if you've had breakfast later, it might not be until between two and four o'clock. Just pay attention to what feels right for you.

Working out at lunchtime can be tricky because you probably won't have time to relax and might increase your Vata because all you've done is go, go, go all day. But if that's the only time you have to exercise, it's better than nothing, and for some people it might be a great way to blow off steam and reduce stress. The point is, if your energy is good, your digestion is strong, and you are healthy, don't change anything. Just try to eat in a quiet setting rather than in front of your computer or while talking on the phone.

Some people need to eat just before they work out; others need to wait at least two hours after a meal before exercising.

If you must work out in the evening, be sure to have a good lunch, with a smaller meal or a snack in the afternoon (and take 2 EPA/DHA or flaxseed oil capsules). Have a postworkout shake on your way home and a lighter dinner with a smaller amount of clean protein, vegetables, spices, good fats, and the amount of carbohydrates that are appropriate for your metabolic profile and weight goals.

Be sure to take your glutamine again before bed.

A TYPICAL DAY FOR HIM AND HER

One problem I encounter almost daily in my practice is that clients, believe it or not, are not consuming *enough* calories. Too often chronic dieters are still trying to lose weight by severely restricting their caloric intake. But, as I've already said, more is not better and neither is less. And in this case, the one thing you absolutely *do not* want to do is reduce your calories too much, which would, in turn, reduce your metabolic rate and sacrifice lean muscle tissue. You need sufficient calories to meet your basal metabolic rate, and if you consistently follow the Ayurvedic pattern of eating a larger lunch, walking, resting, having your midafternoon protein snack and a lighter dinner, you'll burn your calories efficiently, lower your body fat, and increase lean muscle, simply because your digestive system is working efficiently.

Just so you can see how much food you should actually be eating—probably more than you thought and most likely more than you do now—I've worked out a typical day's meal plan for an average "lightly active" (meaning someone who works out fewer than three times a week) female and one for an average, lightly active male. Both these plans are wheat and gluten free (those without gluten sensitivities should feel free to substitute gluten-based grains if they wish), both are low in dairy, and neither contains any starchy carbohydrates. They would be acceptable for any of the three constitutional types, but skinny Vatas could certainly add more good fats and starchy carbs without worrying about their weight. By increasing their level of exercise, this hypothetical male and female would be able to increase their caloric intake as well, and neither of them should be eating any *less* than is recommended here, unless otherwise recommended by a medical or nutrition/fitness professional.

Keep in mind that when we are eating freely, not "on a diet" or "counting calories," we are likely to be consuming more calories on some days than on others, simply because we've been more active or because we're just hungrier. The goal of learning to listen to your body and follow your natural intuition is to become free of obsessive calorie counting. With that in mind, look at the meal plans as guidelines, not as prescriptions to be followed without deviation.

Female, Age 35, 5 ft. 4 in., 140 lb.

Before Workout

1 cup green tea
  with
½ teaspoon fresh lemon juice

¼ ounce fresh ginger

¼ teaspoon honey

½ medium apple with skin, if needed; if not here, have before breakfast

Now work out.

Postworkout Shake

4 tablespoons (20 grams) protein powder
with

2 ounces almond soy, or skim milk

¼ teaspoon cardamom

¼ cup fresh strawberries or 1 teaspoon cocoa powder

6 ounces water

Breakfast

4 ounces 1% fat cottage cheese

¼ teaspoon cinnamon

1 ounce roasted, salted sunflower seeds

1 whole fig, chopped

¼ teaspoon maple syrup

1 tablespoon flaxseed oil

Lunch (Asian)

(Take 2 EPA/DHA or flaxseed oil capsules)

1 cup miso soup

5 ounces baked or broiled salmon fillet (or protein of choice)

1 tablespoon chutney

1 tablespoon wasabi

¼ ounce fresh ginger

2 ounces soy sauce (tamari)

2 cups stir-fried broccoli flowerets

2 cups tossed green salad

1 teaspoon Korean salad dressing

½ navel orange

1 cup herbal tea

Now walk 5 to 10 minutes and rest 5 to 10 minutes.

Afternoon Snack

4 Health Valley or (nongluten) rice crackers
2 ounces Cheddar-style almond cheese or
    goat or sheep's milk cheese
1 cup herbal tea

Dinner

(Take 2 EPA/DHA or flaxseed oil capsules)
1 cup chicken and rice soup
    with
¼ teaspoon fennel seed
¼ teaspoon cumin seed
¼ teaspoon turmeric
¼ teaspoon ginger
¼ teaspoon cinnamon
    or
¼ to ½ teaspoon curry powder
    or
¼ to ½ teaspoon garam masala
    or
a spice blend of your choice
    and
¼ teaspoon sea salt

3 ounces barbecued chicken breast with barbecue sauce
1 cup stir-fried chopped onion
1 cup stir-fried sliced shiitake mushrooms
½ cup steamed, chopped sweet red bell pepper
1 cup chopped kale
    sautéed with
1 teaspoon sesame oil

1 tablespoon chutney
2 yogurt-covered almonds
1 cup chamomile tea

This meal plan provides approximately 1,970 calories: 646 calories
from fat; 96 calories from saturated fat; 149 grams of protein; 200

grams of carbohydrate; 1,154 milligrams of calcium; and 41 grams of dietary fiber. This breaks down to 29 percent of calories from protein; 40 percent from carbohydrates; and 31 percent from fat—only 5 percent of which is from saturated fat. The plan meets all the daily requirements for nutrients recommended by the American Dietetic Association, including those for calcium and fiber, even though these meals are very low in dairy and entirely wheat and gluten free. And remember—this is for a "lightly active" person. The more you work out, the more you get to eat. Just remember to eat that bigger meal at lunch and include some strength training.

Male, Age 35, 6 ft., 180 lb.

Before Workout

1 cup green tea
  with
½ teaspoon fresh lemon juice
¼ ounce fresh ginger
¼ teaspoon honey

½ medium Bartlett pear, or have with breakfast

Now work out.

Postworkout Shake

5 tablespoons (25 grams) protein powder
2 ounces almond soy, or skim milk
¼ teaspoon cardamom
½ cup fresh blueberries or 1 to 2 teaspoons cocoa powder
6 ounces water

Breakfast

2 extra-large scrambled eggs
1 teaspoon olive oil
1 ounce rice mozzarella cheese
2 cups stir-fried spinach
1 tablespoon salsa
2 teaspoons uncooked flaxseed oil
1 cup herbal tea

Lunch

(Take 2 EPA/DHA or flaxseed oil capsules)
1 cup tomato-vegetable soup
6 ounces baked or broiled fresh tuna
1 tablespoon teriyaki sauce with roasted garlic
1 cup stir-fried chopped onion
1 cup stir-fried sliced shiitake mushrooms
1 cup chopped sweet red bell pepper
2 cups stir-fried broccoli flowerets
1 tablespoon chutney
2 cups tossed green salad
1 tablespoon oil and vinegar dressing
¼ ounce crystallized ginger
1 cup herbal tea

Afternoon Snack

1 cup black bean soup
3 ounces jalapeño Jack almond cheese
½ medium apple with skin

Dinner

(Take 2 EPA/DHA or flaxseed oil capsules)
1 cup turkey vegetable soup
   with
¼ teaspoon curry powder

5 ounces roasted boneless turkey breast
3 tablespoons whole cranberry sauce
1 cup chopped onion
1 cup chopped kale
1 cup boiled chopped sweet green bell peppers
1 cup green beans
   stir-fried with
1 teaspoon to 1 tablespoon olive oil
1 teaspoon chutney

2 yogurt-covered almonds
1 cup chamomile tea

This meal plan provides approximately 2,660 calories: 855 calories from fat; 169 calories from saturated fat; 200 grams of protein; 280 grams of carbohydrate; 2,100 milligrams of calcium; and 67 grams of dietary fiber. This breaks down to approximately 30 percent of calories from protein; 40 percent from carbohydrates; and 30 percent from fat—only 6 percent of which is from saturated fat. The plan meets all the daily requirements for nutrients recommended by the American Dietetic Association, including those for calcium and fiber, even though it is very low in dairy and entirely wheat and gluten free. And remember, this is for a "lightly active" person. The more you work out, the more you get to eat.

Now, let's move on to some additional suggestions for meals and snacks that will assure you of getting what you need.

The Best Fuel for Your Constitutional Type

The following meal plans apply to everyone, of all constitutional types. But, as you surely understand by now, exactly how you fulfill your body's need for macronutrients, and how you prepare and flavor your foods, will depend on whether you are a Vata, Pitta, or Kapha, and—even more important—what kind of imbalance you may be experiencing at any given time. So we'll be following up this basic outline with specific suggestions for Vata, Pitta, and Kapha. Make sure you rotate your choices and don't fall into the habit of eating the same thing day after day. One idea that makes it very easy for clients to get more vegetables into their diet is to try to make time twice a week to sautée up a big batch (see sautéed kale recipe page 213). This way you always have vegetables in the fridge ready to add to soups or omelettes or some type of protein. Just heat and add a chutney and you're ready—it takes 2 minutes. Ayurveda believes we should cook fresh every day, but that's just not realistic for many people. Stock up on frozen organic vegetables to use in a pinch—just add a little ghee and chutney to flavor them.

The Basic Meal Plan

Your basic mantra should always be "something warm, something with protein, salads and/or vegetables with good oils, spices, and flavorings, a small sweet for dessert, walk, rest." People who tend to be carbohydrate intolerant, such as Kaphas, type A Pittas, and those who store most of their fat above the waist, should try to eat more proteins, good fats, and vegetables and fewer of the starchy carbohydrates. Vatas can handle more starchy carbohydrates, such as sweet potatoes, squash, even French fries, and they get to have more heavy, oily, grounding foods.

Breakfast

Hot, nongluten cereal with nuts and spices and 3 or 4 ounces of protein, such as cottage cheese or some hard cheese like goat's milk, Cheddar, or almond cheese

> *or*

A 2- or 3-egg omelet cooked in olive oil with non–cow's milk cheese such as almond, feta or other goat's milk, or sheep's milk cheese, and vegetables

> *or*

Nongluten bread such as rice or millet with almond, cashew, or peanut butter, spices such as cinnamon, and a sweetener, such as ½ teaspoon of preserves or maple syrup

> *or*

Cottage cheese with sunflower seeds, almonds, cinnamon, cumin, and a drop of maple syrup

> *or*

A rice or soy or whey protein shake made with 2 to 3 ounces of almond, rice, or soy milk, flavored with cinnamon and cardamom, and 4 to 6 ounces of water (add some cocoa powder if you like)

> *or*

A tofu scramble. Just like an omelet, but made with tofu instead. You can scramble tofu in some olive oil and add spices, rice or almond cheese, and vegetables. It's a perfect meal for a non–meat eater. You can also buy a prepared spice mix called Tofu Scramble by Fantastic to add right to the pan.

With these six menu ideas, you can be sure that you're not eating the same breakfast every day.

Lunch

Soup, such as miso, vegetable, chicken and rice, or black bean. (Soup is warm, low in calories, and high in flavor.) Later in the book I recommend some good-quality organic companies whose products are lower in sodium. Just add extra veggies and spices—these soups are quick, warm, and delicious!

> 4 to 6 ounces of protein, such as fish, organic poultry, or organic meats
>
> > *or*
>
> A nonmeat idea: quinoa or rice and beans with feta, almond, or cottage cheese, or a vegetable burger, or eggs, or tofu
> Salad or sautéed vegetables with olive, sesame, or walnut oil and good flavorings
> Small sweet
> Tea

Morning and Afternoon Snacks

I recommend that you try to eat real food as much as possible (too many people, particularly in the fitness world, actually seem to be living on protein bars instead of food), but if you're really stuck, rather than skip this important meal altogether you can have a protein bar. Just try not to eat too many because they can cause gas and bloating if you overdo them. If you do eat protein bars, try to find the ones I've listed on page 282, which have good EFAs and a good ratio of proteins, fats, and carbs. Let your digestion be your guide.

Organic nuts and seeds and ½ piece of fruit (one of my favorite combinations is to split open a date or fig or pear and add 1 teaspoon almond or cashew butter or tahini—a little goes a long way and the fat and protein in the nut butter balances the sugar in fruit)

or

A cup of soup, 4 ounces of protein (poultry, meat, fish, rice cheese, almond cheese, or feta cheese, or an egg), and vegetables

or

A protein shake (pages 144, 146)

or

Rice bread with nut butter and preserves

Dinner

Soup with additional vegetables and spices
3 to 4 ounces of protein such as fish, chicken, tofu, tempeh, eggs, almond cheese, feta cheese, or cottage cheese
Salad or vegetables sautéed with good oil and flavored with herbs and spices
Up to ½ cup nongluten starch such as squash, sweet potato, quinoa, buckwheat, or basmati rice
Small sweet
Tea

Evening Snack

Warm cow's, soy, rice, or almond milk flavored with cinnamon, cardamom, or cocoa

or

Tea, such as Vata Tea, Celestial Seasonings Sleepytime, Calming Tea by Traditional Medicinal, peppermint, chamomile, or Celestial Seasonings Grandma's Tummy Mint, any of which will be satisfying and calming

With these basic meals plans in mind, you can now tailor the menus to your own constitutional type. Please remember that all these guidelines are meant as suggestions. If something doesn't feel right for you at any particular time, you shouldn't stick with it as if it were written in stone. The point is that once you learn to tune in to your own digestion and energy levels, you'll be able to determine how much of any particular food is good for *you*.

THE PERFECT VATA DAY

These are some basic Ayurvedic recommendations to keep you in balance. Bear in mind you still need to make them specific to your situation. Cooked, warm, soupy, light foods that do not overwhelm the sensitive Vata digestion are best for you. All your foods should be served at room temperature or warmer. Cold salads or foods taken straight from the refrigerator will only intensify your body's tendency to be dry and cold, especially if it's winter or you live in a cold climate. For the same reason, all dry foods should include some protein and good oil and should be lubricated before you eat them. The worst substances for you are caffeine and white sugar, which will aggravate your Vata nervous system and send you flying off the roof. But you do need sweet, sour, and salty tastes in your diet. Substitute honey or another natural sweetener such as maple syrup or Sucanat (pure cane sugar) for the white sugar. And use small quantities of sea salt, which has more trace minerals and better, stronger taste than commercial table salt. Vatas should usually avoid beans (which can leave you gassy and bloated), except for soybeans (tofu). When you do eat beans, prepare them with ghee (clarified butter) or with olive, walnut, or sesame oil, and use mildly warming or carminative (gas-reducing) herbs and spices such as basil, oregano, ginger, cardamom, cinnamon, cumin, coriander, or dill.

The grains that would be most helpful to "taming" your Vata are basmati rice, corn, and quinoa, because they are sweet and lighter to digest than other types of grain, but they should be cooked and served warm, with oils and spices. Other foods that will be beneficial to your digestive health are pumpkin, sesame, and sunflower seeds; almonds; miso; buttermilk; carrots, beets, green leafy vegetables, broccoli, and winter squash, all sautéed in good oil and flavored with

carminative spices; avocado; baked sweet or white potato; and yogurt. Try the recipe for a traditional Ayurvedic mung dahl (page
242); it's a good source of complete protein and is easy for Vatas to
digest.

Avoid apple juice, which is too astringent for you, but go for fresh-
squeezed orange or grapefruit juice, or vegetable juices, all of which
will help your digestion. Other good fruits and juices would be
tomato, pomegranate, carrot, apricot, peach, strawberry, and raspberry.

The animal products that would be best for you are ghee, warm
milk, yogurt, cooked cheese, buttermilk, and organic eggs, as well as
fish and organic, free-range chicken or turkey.

Tailoring the Menus to Balance Vata

You're probably not trying to lose weight, and you need plenty of oil
to keep you lubricated and grounded, as well as sweetness to soothe
your sensitive nervous system, so you should cook your breakfast
omelet in plenty of oil and add a generous amount of cow's or goat's
milk cheese or almond or rice cheese. Use as much nut butter or ghee
as you like on your bread, and sweeten it with maple syrup and cinnamon. Add plenty of nuts, seeds, and cinnamon to your cottage
cheese.

At lunch, make sure you don't forget the warming soup. Opt for
the quinoa or basmati rice and beans, as long as you can digest them.
If you're eating animal protein, make sure it's warm, not straight
from the refrigerator. Choose the sautéed vegetables more often than
cold salads, especially in winter, and make sure you flavor them with
warming, sweet, carminative spices and flavors.

Your snacks, too, should be warm, so try the soup or some warm
protein like scrambled eggs. Stick to the nuts and seeds listed above
for Vatas, and if those are too hard for you to digest, try using nut
butters instead. If you're having a slice of bread, be absolutely sure to
add the nut butter or ghee and cinnamon.

The same guidelines, of course, hold true for dinner. A creamy
soup such as cream of broccoli, asparagus, or mushroom would be
good for you. And, as always, be sure your proteins, vegetables, and
grains are cooked in plenty of good oil and flavored with sweet,
warming, gas-reducing spices and flavors.

The teas that would be best for calming and soothing your Vata are chamomile, Grandma's Tummy Mint (made by Celestial Seasonings), Eater's Digest (Traditional Medicinal), Sleepytime (Celestial Seasonings), Calming Tea (Traditional Medicinal), decaf green tea, and, of course, Vata Tea (Maharishi Ayur-Ved), which is made up of licorice, ginger, cardamom, and cinnamon.

THE PERFECT PITTA DAY

In general, astringent, bitter, and sweet foods are those most suited to the Pitta constitution (which is why those mocha iced coffees are so appealing,) while sour foods are to be avoided and oily, salty, or fried foods should be eaten only in moderation. Honey may be too heating for the fiery Pitta, so it would be best to use moderate amounts of either maple syrup or Sucanat (pure cane sugar) as your sweetener of choice. The best fats for your digestive health are olive oil, coconut oil, and ghee. Sea salt, which has more trace minerals and a stronger taste than regular table salt, is the best kind to use in small quantities. Because you need to balance Pitta's fire, you should stay away from too many "hot" spices such as cloves, mustard, onion, chilies, radish or horseradish, and cayenne. Helpful spices would be ginger, cumin, coriander, fennel, anise, and cardamom, and cinnamon in moderation (its sweetness will curb your cravings, but too much may be overheating), all of which are pungent but also sweet. But listen to your body and don't overdo. Too much dry ginger, for example, might give you a canker sore, and too many acidic fruits (except for limes) and fruit juices could upset your digestion, as will the frequent use of tomatoes, beets, eggplant, corn, carrots, the spicier leafy greens—such as mustard greens—and papayas, all of which are heating. If you are a high Pitta, you may already have noticed that when you eat an Italian meal of pasta with tomato sauce, salad with vinegar, and red wine, for example, you finish the meal feeling hot. The tomatoes, red wine, and vinegar are all "heating" ingredients. Raw onions and garlic might also be too heating for you, but sautéed in oil, they become sweet and may be better for your digestion. Excessive quantities of peanuts and cashews are often too oily for the Pitta's digestion. Try sunflower seeds instead. Alcohol, red meat, shellfish, and caffeine can be major Pitta provokers. Consume them in moderation.

Foods that are good for cooling Pitta's fire are organic milk, cottage cheese, basmati rice, barley, millet, quinoa, cucumber, lettuce, winter squash, yams, tofu, avocado, and sweet fruits such as figs, grapes, raisins, dates, blueberries, red raspberries, peaches, apples, pears, mango, and coconut, all of which are cooling. If you are a type A Pitta/Kapha, you would do best to add digestive spices like fresh ginger, fennel, cumin, coriander, cardamom, or cinnamon to your dairy to help your digestion and still cool you down. Bitter and astringent herbal teas and nonalcoholic beers may also help to cool and calm you.

Tailoring the Menus to Balance Pitta

Flavor your breakfast cereal, cottage cheese, or bread with the sweet taste of maple syrup—just a little bit will do the trick. Cook your omelet in olive oil with some vegetables, use rice, almond, feta, or cow's milk cheese—in rotation—and sweeten the veggies, if you like, with a tablespoon of mango chutney. Use sunflower or pumpkin seeds in your cottage cheese.

For lunch, you'd be better off with eggs, tofu, fish, or organic poultry than with red meat. Have quinoa or basmati rice for their cooling, sweet qualities, but don't overdo the starch, particularly if you're watching your weight. Try a cooling salad made with cucumber, lettuce, and avocado, and use good olive oil in the dressing. The best vegetables for you would be corn, collards, broccoli, kale, red or green chard, onions, red peppers, bok choy, squash, snow peas, celery, or cabbage, sautéed in olive oil or ghee and sweetened with a bit of mild curry or mango chutney.

At snack time, you can have peanuts or nut butter once in a while, but if you're concerned about your weight don't overdo them. Try sunflower seeds instead, or vegetable soup with a quarter pound of protein such as cottage cheese or tuna fish.

Follow the same guidelines at dinner: fish or poultry or tofu; a moderate amount of nongluten grain; a cooling salad dressed with olive oil, or sautéed vegetables flavored with something sweet, and a small sweet to finish the meal.

The best teas for you would be chamomile, peppermint or spearmint, red raspberry, green tea, PMS tea (by Traditional Medicinal), which has dandelion, is cooling, and helps remove excess water, and Pitta Tea (by Maharishi Ayur-Ved), which combines cardamom, licorice, ginger, cinnamon, and dried rose petals and also has a cooling effect.

THE PERFECT KAPHA DAY

You need warming, drying, activating foods and should be avoiding those that are cold, wet, or excessively oily or salty. In addition, you should avoid an excess of dairy products, especially yogurt, because they increase the amount of mucus in the system. *How* you consume dairy is extremely important in Ayurveda. Milk that comes from free-range, antibiotic- and hormone-free animals, and that has been boiled and spiced, is considered more digestible and less Kapha than homogenized milk drunk cold directly from the refrigerator. If you do use oil, make it canola or sesame oil, in small quantities. To control your tendency to gain weight, avoid processed white sugar, which will increase your blood sugar swings and lead to further carbohydrate cravings, but do use honey, which can be warming and helpful for weight reduction (because in addition to being sweet, it is also astringent). That's why I suggest green tea with lemon, ginger, and honey.

For Kaphas, Ayurveda suggests a mostly vegetarian, low-fat diet. Combining that philosophy with the principles of sports nutrition and your own hormonal profile, you would probably do best obtaining the bulk of your fiber and carbohydrates from the least starchy sources or those that are lowest on the glycemic index, which would be vegetables and salads. Stay away from too much rice, pasta, and potatoes, and if you do eat grains, try whole nongluten grains such as millet, quinoa, buckwheat, basmati rice, and brown rice, which are less Kapha. Then add some good proteins such as tofu, fish, or lean organic poultry, eggs, or beans and quinoa, and moderate quantities of good fats and oils. And don't forget your EFAs, which will help to lower your Kapha body fat.

Your foods should be cooked with spices such as cayenne, cinnamon, ginger, black pepper, mustard, cloves, celery seed, dill, curry or garam masala—in other words, those that are spicy, heating, stimulating, and drying. You might also try onions and shiitake mushrooms sautéed in a moderate amount of good olive oil. Dark leafy greens will also dry you out and get you moving, as will spiced, cooked fruits and cranberry, pomegranate, carrot, grapefruit, and green vegetable juices, in moderation. Stay away from cooling, heavy fruits like bananas, dates, mangoes, apples, and apple juice. If you can't give them up altogether, do remember to use them sparingly.

Herbal teas that are pungent, bitter, and astringent can be helpful to the Kapha digestion. Try Eater's Digest, Be Trim, ginger tea, green tea, or Kapha Tea, made up of cinnamon, cloves, cardamom, ginger, and black pepper.

Tailoring the Menus to Balance Kapha

Use warming ginger or cinnamon in your breakfast cereal, on your cottage cheese, and on your rice bread. Use honey as your sweetener. Try rice, almond, or feta cheese in your omelet (they are less Kapha than cow's milk cheeses and therefore don't congest the system as much), add some chopped spinach or kale and cook the omelet in a small quantity of canola oil. Go easy on the nut butter; too much would be detrimental to the already sluggish Kapha metabolism.

Warm soup is important for you at lunchtime, so don't forget it. Eat plenty of warm, bitter leafy greens, and flavor them with garlic, curry, garam masala, black pepper, dill, or spicy salsas. If you do use animal protein, stick to fish or lean organic poultry. Other good proteins for you would be eggs or beans and quinoa.

A cup of warming vegetable soup would be a good snack for you, along with four ounces of one of the proteins just mentioned.

It's particularly important for sluggish Kaphas to keep their evening meal light, so stick to fish and, again, plenty of vegetables with warming, drying spices and flavors.

GIVE YOURSELF A LUNCH BREAK

I'm sure you're beginning to understand by now how important it is for you to try to eat your main meal in the middle of the day and to do so in a relaxing and calm environment so that your body will be able to devote its energies to digestion rather than the telephone or the computer. And you also know why it's equally important to take a short walk (to get things moving) and then rest briefly before going on with your day. This is the biggest challenge for my clients, but the one that makes the most difference.

In the frenetic world most of us inhabit, however, it's sometimes difficult to do this, particularly if you're eating lunch at your desk. Even a closed office door isn't necessarily a deterrent to people who feel they must talk to you *right now,* and the telephone simply doesn't understand the principles of Ayurveda. For these reasons, I tell my clients that if at all possible, they should take the time to actually *go out to lunch.* Not only will this assure you of getting the break you need, but also, in many locations throughout the country, there are local, inexpensive restaurants offering a variety of ethnic cuisines that will provide you with the variety that is so important to keeping your taste buds happy and your cravings under control.

To help you with your choices, I've listed below five different ethnic cuisines with menu choices that would be appropriate for Vata, Pitta, and Kapha.

Japanese

Soup: Miso or vegetable soup, good for Vata, Pitta, and Kapha.

Protein: Salmon, chicken, or shrimp, good for Vata, Pitta, and Kapha. Tofu, okay for Vata, Pitta, and Kapha. Vatas and Kaphas may need to add gas-reducing spices such as ginger.

Salad: Good for Pitta and Kapha with ginger dressing. May be too cool for Vatas, who could add a creamy dressing with sesame oil.

Sautéed Vegetables: Good for all types. Lots of greens for Pitta and Kapha; less for Vatas.

Rice: ½ to 1 cup is okay for Vatas; Pittas and Kaphas don't really need it.

Dessert: Either ½ orange or a piece of crystallized ginger would be good for all three types.

Beverage: Green tea with ginger is good for all three types; Vatas should ask for decaf. Peppermint tea would be great for all types.

Spices: Wasabi, ginger, and soy sauce are okay for all three types. Pittas should go lighter on the wasabi and soy, which can be heating.

Mexican

Soup: Black bean okay for Pitta and Kapha. Vatas would do better with vegetable.

Burrito: Okay for Vatas. All types should try to rotate wheat with nongluten grains, or eliminate wheat and gluten for a period of time. Ask for a "naked burrito"—rice, beans, and vegetables with salsa, guacamole, and sour cream without the tortilla wrapper. Vata and Pitta can use more guacamole and sour cream than Kapha. Pitta should not use "hot" salsa—try using mild. Kaphas can use more hot salsa. Additional protein for all types can be fish, tofu (if available,) shrimp, or chicken, or a combination of black beans and rice.

Fajita: Great for all types. Use the proteins recommended for burritos. Add sautéed vegetables, sour cream, guacamole, and salsa in amounts recommended above. As with the burrito, ask them to "hold the wrapper" and give you extra vegetables instead.

Rice: Small amounts for Pitta and Kapha. Vatas can use more.

Dessert: ½ a piece of fruit or a small portion of flan. A little should be enough if you've had a good meal. Kaphas, however, should try to stick to the fruit.

Beverage: Lemonade is good for Vatas. Pittas might want herbal iced tea, and Kaphas can have regular iced tea.

Spices: Cumin, oregano, thyme, cinnamon, and allspice are good for all three types. Pittas should go easier on the heating spices and add more cooling avocado or salad. Kaphas can go to town on the picante sauce and jalapeños.

Thai

Soup: Clear vegetable for Kapha; tom yum kha, or lemongrass and coconut milk with basil and chilies, for Pitta and Vata. (The lemongrass and coconut will balance the spice of the chilies for Pittas.)

Protein: Shrimp, tofu, chicken, or fish are good for all three types.

Vegetable: Lots, for all types. Kaphas would do well with the red curry sauces, which are hotter. Pittas might do better with coconut green curry sauces, which are milder and sweeter. Vatas are fine with either type.

Salad: Good for Pitta and Kapha. Might be too cold for Vata.

Jasmine rice: More for Vata; smaller quantities for Pitta and Kapha.

Dessert: A small amount of ginger or green tea ice cream would be good for Vatas and Pittas. (If you're with a friend, split dessert.) Kaphas should stick with a piece of fruit.

Beverage: Decaf Thai iced tea, which is very sweet, would be good for Vata and Pitta. Kapha can have decaf Thai iced coffee or tea.

Spices: Ginger, basil, mint, tamarind, chilies, lemongrass.

Indian

Soup: Vegetable, lentil, and mung dahl are good for all three types.

Protein: Tandoori shrimp, tofu, chicken, or fish are good for all three types.

Vegetable: Any of the wide variety available, with lots of spices and flavors. Good for all three types. Creamed spinach dishes with cheeses are good for Vata and Pitta. Kaphas should probably stick to the lighter sautéed vegetables.

Rice: ½ to 1 cup of basmati rice would be good for Pittas and Vatas. Pittas should stick with the smaller amount, Vatas can have more. Kaphas should stay away from the rice and eat more of the vegetables.

Dessert: Kir or Indian rice pudding (which is wonderful with milk, almonds, cardamom, and raisins) are okay for Vata and Pitta. A bite of kir or mango-ginger ice cream won't hurt a Kapha, but a piece of fruit would be better.

Beverage: Lassis are good for Vatas, mango lassis for Pittas. Chai would be good for all three types; Kaphas should ask for skim milk, if possible. Some chais are spicier, using more cloves and black pepper—better for Kaphas, but sweeter is better for Pittas. Vatas and Pittas should try to get decaf beverages.

Spices: Southern Indian cooking is more heating than that of northern India. Pittas should stick to the milder spices and use more mango or lime chutneys. Vatas and Kaphas can use more of the heating spices.

American

Soup: Clear vegetable, chicken and rice, or split pea, among the many choices, would be good for all three types. Creamy vegetable soups are good for Vatas and okay for Pittas, but Kaphas should stick with clear.

Protein: Fish, tofu, organic chicken or turkey, shrimp, and other seafood are good for all three types. Try to rotate proteins for best digestion.

Vegetable: All kinds of sautéed vegetables are good for all three types. Try flavoring them with chutney, lemon, or olive oil.

Salad: Good for Pitta and Kapha, but may be too cold for Vatas, particularly in fall and winter. Pittas and Kaphas should use olive oil dressings; Vatas would do well with sesame oil, or ranch, blue cheese, or another "creamy" dressing.

Potatoes and grain: All types should try to alternate gluten with nongluten grains. More potatoes and grains are okay for Vatas. Pittas can have up to ½ cup of nongluten grain. Kaphas should try sticking with extra salad or vegetables instead of the grain, if possible.

Dessert: 2 yogurt-covered almonds, a piece of crystallized ginger, or a small piece of good chocolate would be fine for all types.

Beverage: Eater's Digest tea, peppermint tea, or decaffeinated coffee are fine for all types, and you'll be amazed how satisfying peppermint tea with honey can be.

Spices: Make sure your meal includes all six tastes and qualities for satisfaction and good digestion.

A SPICY VARIETY

Remember that the key is to try to include all the tastes and qualities of foods at every meal and to "listen to your body" so that you will be able to keep it in balance. If you're a Pitta/Vata, for example, some sour taste like lemon in water will help to increase your digestive fire, but too much may aggravate your Pitta. You'll know if you've gone overboard because the reaction of your body—perhaps developing a canker sore—will tell you when it's time to cut back.

Now that you know when, how much, and what to eat, and you're aware of the importance of trying to relax while you eat for maximum digestion and exercising for mobilizing body fat and reducing stress, you're set to begin a satisfying, adventurous, and health-promoting culinary adventure. I hope you're going to find it as exciting and rewarding as I did when I first discovered the benefits of integrating the wisdom of Ayurveda with the science of Western nutrition.

Part Two

A Simple Action Plan

CHAPTER EIGHT

Getting It Moving

A Simple Cleanse to Get Rid of the Toxins and Get You Going

By now I hope you've been able to determine your constitutional type and understand imbalances; you should be more familiar with which foods, herbs, and spices will help to maximize your digestion, and you're hopefully more aware of what ratio of proteins, fats, and carbohydrates will keep you in balance, so that you can mobilize body fat, develop lean muscle, and arrive at your desired weight. Before you begin your newfound balanced approach to eating and health, however, it's a good idea to start with a gentle internal "spring cleaning." Ayurveda and traditional Chinese medicine both recommend that you cleanse a minimum of twice a year, at the change of seasons. But cleansing is also a good way to jump-start your new program in order to achieve the best results in the shortest period of time. In my practice (and at the gym) I see many fitness enthusiasts who are perpetually overdoing the whey protein, supplements, and energy bars. Once again, more is not always better. Sometimes your body just needs a break, and as I keep reiterating, symptoms like gas and bloating, swollen glands, skin irritations, allergies, or sinus problems are usually signs that toxins are building up in the system.

While ideally our bodies are designed to rid themselves of toxins, there is extensive evidence, as reported by Dr. Mark Percival in his article "Nutritional Support for Detoxification," published in *Applied Nutritional Science Reports,* that the overload of environmental toxins in our modern world may require that we provide our systems with some help in this area.

My own first experience with cleansing was through meeting Pamela Serure, the author of two books on cleansing, *The Three Day Energy Fast* and *Three Days to Vitality,* and the previous owner of Get Juiced in Bridgehampton, New York. I went through her program as part of my research for the Peninsula Spa, spending three days at the beach with my bicycle and my books. I lived on lovely, fresh, organic fruit and vegetable juices. I slept, I read, I walked on the beach, I sat in the steamroom, and at the end of those three days I was exploding with energy, my skin was clear and radiant, and my stomach was nice and calm and flat.

There are many different ways to do a cleanse, and when I moved to Colorado, I learned that Ayurveda recommends a seasonal cleanse called *pancha karma* to purify and strengthen the physical body. But this is a rather in-depth system of cleansing that should not be undertaken without the supervision of a qualified Ayurvedic practitioner. The cleanse I recommend here is a bit more Westernized, simpler to implement, and manageable for most people.

Before you start this or any other cleanse, however, you should always check with your personal health care provider to be sure that there is nothing in the program that might exacerbate any underlying health condition you might have.

THE IMPORTANCE OF SEASONAL CHANGE

According to Ayurveda, eating with the seasons is an essential component of listening to your body and understanding its nutritional needs. You'll remember that each of the three constitutional types—Vata, Pitta, and Kapha—is associated with a particular season.

Fall into winter is the Vata time of year. Animals put on heavier coats, and humans add body fat and store additional mucus in the lymphatic system for insulation. As spring (Kapha) and summer (Pitta) approach, we no longer need the excess mucus. As the weather warms up, our internal heat, or Pitta, increases and can become trapped in the system by the mucus that has been building up to keep us warm since the previous fall. You may already have noticed that this is when you begin to suffer from allergies and sinus infections or congestion problems, your digestion might be off, you might feel bloated and uncomfortable, and your skin might break out. All these reactions are simply ways your body is telling you it's full of toxins or excess mucus and heat that need to escape. It's asking for help! Think of your cleanse as a spring cleaning for your body.

The same holds true as summer turns to fall, which is, again, the Vata time of year. As you enter the season associated with the elements of air and ether, you may be feeling a bit more "spacey" and overwhelmed than usual. Ayurveda compares this to wind blowing on a fire. You've probably collected a bit of extra heat in your system during the summer months, which may show up as skin irritations, digestive problems, or even increased PMS or menopausal symptoms. As the cold weather sets in, you'll be accumulating more mucus, which may leave you with a feeling of heaviness. You may even come down with a head cold.

If you look to nature, you'll see that the plants and animals look different. Even our supermarkets don't look the same as they did in the summer. The strawberries and watermelon are gone, their places taken by heavier, warming foods like nuts, sweet potatoes, and squash. These changes should signal you that it's time to add more warm foods and good, monounsaturated oils to your diet. But first, a gentle cleanse can help to detoxify your body, alleviate your symptoms, and ground you for the coming winter.

A cleanse should be relaxing and self-indulgent. It should be looked upon not as a time of deprivation, but as a way of being kind to yourself. I suggest you plan your cleanse by creating a kind of spa weekend for yourself. Take the time to disappear from society for at least the first and second day, or all three days if possible; plan to have a massage or take a yoga class. A steam or a sauna will help to relax you and will also help to pull the toxins out of your lymphatic system. Use a dry brush to brush your skin before you shower in the morning and again before bedtime to stimulate the lymphatic system, mobilize cellulite and body fat, and get rid of the dead cells. Your skin is actually your body's largest detoxifying organ, and if you have built up layers of dead cells and are living in a dry, cold climate, it will be more difficult for accumulated toxins to leave your body.

That's why it's important to get rid of the dead, dry cells so that new ones can grow and your natural oils can get out and not cause additional breakouts. Dry brushing will help to relax your muscles, increase your circulation, even improve your digestion. As an added bonus, your skin should take on a new, youthful glow. You can also treat yourself and your skin to the pampering, soothing, and rejuvenating application of pure oil, like grape seed or almond, which are wonderful for all three constitutional types; cooling coconut oil if you're a Pitta; or warming sesame oil for Vatas and Kaphas. Then add a few drops of essential oils such as lemon, sandalwood, lavender, or another of your choice.

The purpose of these three days* is to help clear all the caffeine, wheat, glutens, and sugar out of the digestive tract, so you might want to try to "clean up your act" a few days before you begin—it really wouldn't be a good idea to go straight from a diet of Big Macs and martinis to eating nothing solid at all. Eat more fresh fruits and vegetables; cut down on animal protein; eat more fish, tofu, rice, and beans, so that the cleanse will not come as such a shock to your system. And remember, it will be a gentle cleanse, not a weekend of torture. Not only will you be drinking plenty of juices, broths, teas, and warm water with lemon, but you'll be taking a variety of nutritional supplements that will help increase the efficacy of the cleanse while providing essential nutrients.

Before you start, you'll need to do a bit of preparatory shopping. Here's a list of things you'll need to have on hand.

---

* Pitta and Kapha constitutional types should follow the program described here for three days (remember that it takes about this long for food to travel through your system, from one end to the other). For small, thin Vatas, however, the cleanse should last just one day, because Vatas simply don't have enough body fat or the strength to go the full three days. Ayurveda also suggests one-day cleanses or "fasts" from solid food for digestive problems and weight management, but not on only water or fruit juice. Do not do the three full days more than twice a year, in spring and in fall—you don't want to slow down your metabolism, you want to clean out your digestive tract.

SHOPPING LIST FOR CLEANSE

Buy organic whenever possible!

For full explanations of the supplements recommended on this list, please see chapter 9. If you have a problem finding any of the items on this list, you can e-mail us at info@thebalancedapproach.com (or see pages 299–315).

Fresh lemons
Honey
Fresh ginger
Fresh fruit: apples, pears, watermelon, berries, etc.
Naturade Aloe Vera Detox Formula
Liquid chlorophyll
Triphala tablets (Planetary Herbs)
Organic (Knudsen's or Mountain Sun) cranberry nectar or apple juice or grape juice
Red Clover Supreme (Gaia Herbs)

> *and*

Scudders Supreme (Gaia Herbs)

> *or*

Milk thistle capsules or tablets (Solgar or Nature's Way)
Herbal teas: green tea, peppermint, chamomile, Grandma's Tummy Mint, Eater's Digest, CCF tea (cumin, coriander, fennel), etc. (see page 263)
Ultra Clear Rice Protein (Metagenics)*
Almond (Blue Diamond) or rice milk (fortified with vitamins A and D and calcium)

---

* Ultra Clear Rice Protein, made by Metagenics, is a rice protein specially designed for cleansing. It contains liver-supportive nutrients, vitamins, and minerals and must be bought through a practitioner such as a nutritionist, chiropractor, or a naturopathic physician. You can check our Web site for more information (see page 306), or you can use any organic rice protein, which can be found at a health food store.

Spices: cardamom, cinnamon, curry, garam masala, rose petal conserve (Maharishi), cumin, coriander, fennel seeds and powder, and turmeric

Lots of vegetables: onions, shiitake mushrooms, kale, broccoli, cabbage, spinach, etc.

Health Valley organic vegetable broth

Probiotic supplement (Metagenics Ultra Flora Dairy Free, or PB8, Jarrow, or New Chapter from a health food store)

Long-handled dry-skin brush

Body oils: grape seed, almond, coconut, or sesame

Essential oils: lavender, lemon, sandalwood, valor, etc.

DOING THE CLEANSE

Make sure that you start the first day as a spa day. Don't try to do this on a crazy, busy day at work.

On the first morning of your cleanse, you'll wake up and drink two cups of warm water or green tea with lemon, honey, and fresh ginger. This combination is weight reducing, and it helps to clear the *ama,* or undigested food particles, and toxins from the system. The honey, in addition to being sweet, is an astringent and will help "scrape" any accumulated toxins from the walls of your colon and stimulate weight loss. The ginger, as you know, is one of the best herbs for removing *ama* and other toxins from the system and will act to stimulate and reinforce the actions of the other herbs. Triphala is a toning Ayurvedic herb made from a combination of three fruits that strengthen the bowels and help to cleanse the system without adding bulk or causing irritation. Then you'll have what I call my Green Drink, comprising aloe vera juice, liquid chlorophyll, and other medicinal herbs mixed with organic cranberry, apple, or grape juice (my own preference is cranberry), to help cleanse the liver and lymphatic system. Throughout the morning, you'll be drinking more warm water with lemon, green tea, herbal teas, and diluted organic fruit juices.

Then, to keep your blood sugar stable and to boost phase two of the detoxification of the liver, you'll have a protein drink made up of protein powder mixed with warm water and almond milk with various spices and flavorings added for taste. In the afternoon, you'll have a large vegetable juice drink including parsley, celery, kale, cucumber, spinach, beets, and a small amount of carrot, as a way to "bathe" the inside of your body in antioxidants.

The juice will be followed by a second protein shake, and you can also have as much warm water with lemon, or herbal tea, as you like. Sipping warm water helps to cleanse the lymphatic system; cold water isn't as effective for this.

In the late afternoon and evening, you'll have a potassium broth—a vegetable soup made up of any combination of sautéed vegetables, such as broccoli, onion, kale, spinach, mushrooms, any other green vegetables you like, and sea salt. This is a warm and satisfying broth that helps to replace the electrolytes and fiber in your system and also adds antioxidants.

You can, if you wish, have a third protein shake. Add more triphala and herbs in the evening, when you'll also add a probiotic supplement of acidophilus, bifidus, and additional good bacteria to replenish the good bacteria in the colon. (As I've discussed, most of us have been overexposed to antibiotics over the course of a lifetime—not only because they've been prescribed for various illnesses, but also from the meat and dairy products in our diet that have been treated with antibiotics. As a result, we have not enough good bacteria in our colon and an overgrowth of candida and yeast that can adversely affect our immune system.)

You'll then be repeating the program over the following two days. As you see, you'll be drinking continuously throughout the day, so you won't be starving.

Here's the whole formula for the cleanse, with all the right ingredients and proportions:

Jennifer's Gentle Juice Cleanse

The evening before you start

2 to 4 triphala tablets (Planetary Formulas)

Your bowels should move during a cleanse; you want to move things out, not have them back up. Start by taking 2; if you don't see results the next morning, up the dose to 4. Your bowels should move without discomfort.

Morning

2 cups warm water or green tea with lemon, honey, and 1 or 2 slices of fresh ginger

2 to 4 triphala tablets (Planetary Formulas)

Green Drink:

1 tablespoon Naturade Aloe Vera Detox Formula (contains milk thistle, burdock, and yellow dock, all of which help to cool and cleanse the liver and are gentle blood purifiers)

1 tablespoon liquid chlorophyll (helps to cleanse the colon and purify the blood)

2 droppers Red Clover Supreme (Gaia Herbs; a gentle blood purifier that is helpful for the liver and lymphatic system)

>   *and*

2 droppers Scudders Supreme (Gaia Herbs; for cleansing the tissues and lymphatic system)

>   *or* (if you can't find the Gaia products)

2 droppers or 1 to 2 capsules milk thistle extract (follow manufacturer's directions)

>   *mixed with*

3 to 4 ounces organic apple, cranberry, or grape juice

Nine A.M.

Protein Shake: (The purpose of the protein shakes is to keep your blood sugar from crashing and to support the liver so that it can perform its detoxifying function properly. The protein shakes are imperative. I usually recommend that people use rice protein and avoid whey or soy on a cleanse.)

FOR FALL AND FOR VATAS AND KAPHAS:

2 scoops Metagenics Ultra Clear Rice Protein or Organic Rice Protein

4 ounces *warm* water

3 ounces almond milk

3 to 4 fresh berries *or* 1 to 2 teaspoons cocoa powder

¼ teaspoon cinnamon

¼ teaspoon cardamom

or

FOR SPRING AND FOR PITTAS:
2 scoops Metagenics Ultra Clear Rice Protein
4 ounces *cool* water
3 ounces almond milk
3 to 4 fresh berries *or* 1 to 2 teaspoons cocoa powder
1 teaspoon Maharishi brand rose petal conserve (optional—this will add sweetness and is good for lowering Pitta and calming the heart)
¼ teaspoon cinnamon
¼ teaspoon cardamom
Add ice and blend

Drink more warm water with lemon and honey, herbal teas, and fruit juices diluted with spring water and lemon or lime throughout the morning. Kaphas may not need to drink as much as other types because they already hold water. Warm water with lemon, ginger, and honey; green tea; and ginger tea are good for lowering Kapha.

Twelve P.M.

Repeat Ultra Clear Protein Shake

Afternoon

Fresh, organic vegetable juices:
8 to 16 ounces of parsley, celery, cucumber, spinach, kale, carrot, and beet combined (if this tastes too bitter, you can add apple and ginger for sweetness)

If possible, get freshly made, organic vegetable juice from a health food store, a juice bar, a spa, or a gym.

Continue to drink more warm water with lemon and honey and more herbal teas throughout the afternoon.

Three to four P.M.

Repeat Ultra Clear Protein Shake

Late Afternoon and Evening

Potassium Broth/Soup: Jennifer's Quick and Easy Version

Use 1 can or ½ carton of Health Valley, Pacific, or any other organic vegetable broth. Simply chop and sauté in olive oil such vegetables as broccoli, kale, spinach, cabbage, carrots, onions, shiitake mushrooms (used in Chinese medicine to support the immune system), and add them to heated vegetable broth along with 1 teaspoon sea salt and spices of choice. Curry, garam masala, cumin, and turmeric work best.

These broths are important for keeping your electrolytes in balance. It's not necessary to puree the vegetables. In fact, they will add fiber along with vitamins and minerals.

Evening

2 to 4 triphala tablets
2 droppers Red Clover Supreme (liver)

> *and*

2 droppers Scudders Supreme (lymph)

> *or*

2 droppers or 1 to 2 capsules milk thistle extract

> *mixed into*

3 to 4 ounces warm water or herbal tea
2 probiotic supplement tablets (Metagenics Ultra Flora Dairy Free)

WHAT TO EXPECT

The reason it's important to make the first day of your cleanse a "spa" day is that you may be a bit cranky and irritable (not the best day to make a good impression on someone who doesn't know you very well!), you may be a bit headachy, even a bit nauseated or tired, and your skin may break out. But these symptoms are simply indications that toxins are already beginning to leave your system. That's why a facial or massage can be so beneficial.

You should think of it as a good thing, but cleansing means that you will, nevertheless feel a little worse before you begin to feel better, and you should expect to rest and take a nap. Try to have the kids go to friends or relatives. Rent a happy movie. Take a walk in the park, write in a journal, do a light workout or take a yoga class, have a massage or a steam or at least a nice hot bath. It's important to fill this day with good things.

The second day is usually marked by ups and downs; your mood may swing from cranky to calm and back again. Try not to plan too many activities on this day. And, again, a little self-indulgence would be beneficial.

On the third day you should be feeling pretty good—your stomach should be a little flatter and your energy should be on the rise, but you might need some extra sleep, so plan to take a nap and give yourself a rest.

By the fourth day you should feel *amazing!* Your eyes should be clearer, your skin will be glowing from all those vegetables, your energy should be up, and you'll be ready to rock and roll!

If you've never done this before, and if your diet has been really bad, it's going to be a bit more difficult the first time. As your body gets healthier and stronger and you begin to eat better-quality foods with more variety and less wheat, gluten, and processed sugar, you can do the cleanse again at the next change of season. Your body will actually look forward to it. As I mentioned, Ayurveda recommends cleansing or "fasting" (but not just on water or juice) one day a week for weight loss, to decrease Kapha, or for digestive problems. You can give it a try—your body might really like it, but, again, don't do three days in a row more than twice a year—it's not necessary.

AFTER THE CLEANSE

After the cleanse, you'll be going back to eating. You'll be ready to start treating your body to the pleasures of eating clean protein, good fats, and nongluten carbohydrates, and you'll be able to stop your cravings by flavoring your food with delicious herbs and spices. You probably won't be craving an extra-large pizza anyway, because by now your body knows what feels good and what doesn't. To continue the cleanse on a deeper level, it is necessary to keep taking the Red Clover Supreme and Scudders Supreme (or the milk thistle if you've been using that instead) for another two weeks or until the bottles are empty. You can also continue to take the triphala for two to four months, five days on and two days off. It's a tonic herb that helps to tone the bowels and remove excess mucus from the colon, and it becomes more beneficial the longer you use it.

Now, make a list of the foods you want to try first, go to your local health food store or supermarket, and begin to reap the rewards of eating the Ayurvedic way.

CHAPTER NINE

Supplementing Your Diet

Too often, as I've seen in my practice, the American tendency to believe that if something is good, more must be better carries over from diet to dietary supplements as well. I can't tell you how often new clients come in literally carrying shopping bags full of supplements. But both Ayurveda and traditional Chinese medicine take the approach that supplements are to be used just as their name implies—as *supplementary* to diet.

Eric Serrano, M.D., a well-known, board-certified family medicine physician, sports nutritionist, and consultant to elite athletes, has pointed out that it is important to eat a normal, varied diet of real food and protein sources, that we should *vary* our protein sources to *maximize* digestion, and that we should use supplements wisely, so as not to miss out on a variety of nutrients. Needless to say, it did my heart good to see even this voice from the medical and fitness worlds starting to look at the role of digestion in overall health as well as the importance of variety in diet.

Having said that, however, I should add that it's equally important to ensure that your diet is not deficient in essential nutrients. I don't think it's a good idea to take megadoses of any single vitamin or mineral unless you are instructed to do so by your own health care practitioner for a specific condition, such as pregnancy or a heart condition. Many vitamins and minerals have either synergistic or antagonistic interactions—too much zinc, for example, inhibits the absorption of copper. And, in fact, we do best when we receive a variety of nutrients from a variety of sources. Studies have shown, for example, that we need a variety of carotenoids derived from foods of different colors—such as strawberries, blueberries, and oranges, as well as carrots. But until recently, multivitamin supplements have provided only one of the carotenoids, beta-carotene. That's now been changed, so that if you look at a bottle of vitamins from a reputable company, you'll see that it contains "mixed carotenoids." This example, however, indicates our tendency to isolate one or two nutrients and depend upon or emphasize them while ignoring others that may be equally important to health.

On the other hand, I do think that many people could benefit from a good blended multivitamin formula, just to be sure they are getting adequate quantities of all the basic nutrients (for recommendations see page 191). In most cases, it would be wise to have your diet analyzed by a professional—preferably a nutritionist/dietitian with a background in sports nutrition or complementary medicine—to determine your particular needs. In this area, as with everything we've discussed so far, I find the Ayurvedic philosophy to make the most sense. When determining what dietary supplements would be appropriate for you, you need to ask, as you do for diet and exercise, "for whom, under what conditions, in what season, at what time of life?"

THERMOGENIC SUPPLEMENTS—APPROPRIATE OR NOT?

When it comes to supplements that are intended to promote weight loss, the approach taken by Ayurveda, traditional Chinese medicine, and Eastern herbalism again differs from that taken by Western fitness and medical practitioners. Too often, fat-burning, thermogenic, stimulating herbs are prescribed immediately, without first determining why a person is heavy or if he or she has recently gained weight as opposed to being heavy from birth.

If the person is genetically heavy or overweight (a Kapha constitutional type), born to heavy parents, a thermogenic, stimulating, fat-burning formula might indeed be appropriate, depending on stress level and adrenal health. If, on the other hand, we are looking at a type A Pitta who is in a Vata emotional imbalance because he or she is overstressed and has been eating too many sweet, sour, salty, or heavy, oily, warm foods for nurturance, that formula would be totally inappropriate. Because, as you now know, overconsumption of the sweet, starchy, heavy foods that soothe the fiery Pitta and calm a Vata imbalance can also throw the body into a Kapha physical imbalance and increase body fat. But heating up and stimulating the Pitta system even further in an effort to burn off the fat could easily exacerbate the problem and put even more stress on already exhausted adrenal glands, leading to yet more cravings for sweet, heavy, grounding foods and to additional weight gain. A qualified herbalist would analyze the Pitta individual and blend a formula that would not put more stress on the adrenal glands, but rather would support them, as well as the liver and the colon, to help the body detoxify and mobilize the fat. It would include a component to heat up and dry out the fat, but that component would be combined with other ingredients that were intended to restore *balance* over the long term. There would be anywhere from one to three herbs in the formula that were directly related to the immediate problem, be it weight gain, congestion, or liver toxicity. The mixture would also contain a carrier herb to deliver the benefits of the first three, and additional herbs to help balance digestion and aid elimination would also be included in the formula. The Eastern approach is based on the belief that nature put plants on the earth to keep the planet in balance and that different plants have an affinity for different organs— gingko for the brain and milk thistle for the liver, to give just two examples—and that plants and herbs, when used properly, can have powerful healing effects.

In the course of my practice, I've sent many clients to herbalists who have helped them not only to lose weight, but also to maximize digestion, support the liver and nervous system, and even, when appropriate, get off antidepressants or nourish their exhausted bodies. Herbal medicine is about nurturing the system back into balance, not about suppressing symptoms or increasing deprivation.

An Example of East vs. West

Ephedra: This is the herb that has probably received more negative publicity than it deserves because it has been misused by athletes to burn fat. It is thermogenic, which means that it helps to stimulate the system and decrease mucus and body fat. It is also a broncho-dilator and is usually included in decongestant formulas for asthma, bronchitis, and other lung disorders. It is a strong stimulant and promotes increased awareness and energy. Taken alone, or in combination with caffeine and other stimulants, however, it can be extremely counterproductive for the typical type A, overweight American. In traditional Chinese medicine and Ayurveda it would never be given alone or combined only with other stimulants, such as green tea or caffeine. Their combination increases Pitta but also puts additional strain on the adrenal glands and increases Vata and adrenaline output. Instead, for a Kapha-imbalanced person who needs to lose weight or decrease congestion or mucus, it would be blended in a formula with adrenal support, digestive herbs, and something to buffer the intensity of its effects. Even Charles Poliquin, the Olympic strength-training coach, has stated that he rarely recommends thermogenics to his clients unless they have an extremely sluggish, Kapha metabolism; otherwise, he sees better fat-loss results from L-glutamine (page 186) and essential fatty acids (page 188). The point is that no one herb or supplement is inherently good or bad. The key is knowing how to use them, who they are for, and under what conditions.

SOME FAVORITE SUPPLEMENTS

This section will first describe a variety of basic supplements that might be appropriate for you in particular circumstances and then make suggestions for a basic regimen that I would recommend to the average person who is neither an extreme athlete nor suffering from any specific or extraordinary deficiency or health problem.

Before going further, I just want to reiterate that I am a nutritionist, not a certified herbalist or a doctor, and although I am familiar and work with all the products on these lists on a regular basis, I always recommend that anyone with any kind of health condition seek the advice of his or her own health care practitioner. Herbs and food are considered medicine in Ayurveda. Any individual can have an allergy or sensitivity to virtually any food or herb. Please use this information with care and find a qualified practitioner to guide you in using these products.

None of these products or the statements about them has been evaluated by the Food and Drug Administration, and the products are not intended to diagnose, treat, care for, or prevent disease. They are presented here as suggestions for better nutrition only, not as medical advice. Pregnant or lactating women or anyone with allergies or who is taking any medication should consult his or her health care practitioner or primary care physician before using any supplement. Always read labels carefully, especially if a product is new to you, and heed all directions and cautions.

Ayurvedic Products

Teas

Teas provide a very gentle, effective way to use herbs. They can be soothing or cooling or stimulating, depending on the herb or the blend that is used. All these teas, made by the Maharishi Ayur-Ved Company, are available at most health food stores. If you can't find them, you can visit our Web site at www.thebalancedapproach.com for more information.

Vata Tea: A calming, soothing tea made of licorice, ginger, cardamom, and cinnamon, to de-stress your nervous system. Sip it throughout the day, especially in a hectic environment.

Pitta Tea: Made up of cardamom, licorice, ginger, cinnamon, and dried rose petals, this soothing tea will cool you down when you're hot, irritable, or impatient or simply when the weather is hot. The rose petals have a wonderful, cooling effect on the body and are soothing to the heart.

Kapha Tea: This tasty, spicy blend of cinnamon, cloves, cardamom, ginger, and black pepper is heating and stimulating and will help to decrease both body fat and mucus in the system.

Be Trim tea: A blend of mint, fennel, Indian kino, *Gymnema sylvestre,* manjista, cinnamon, cardamom, black pepper, long pepper, turmeric, rose petal, and licorice, this tea is heating but not stimulating and is designed to curb and balance the appetite as well as to slow the absorption of carbohydrates, decrease body fat, and balance cholesterol metabolism. I have seen it work wonders with my clients in helping to manage cravings.

Ayurvedic Herbs Gaining Popularity in the Fitness World

Ashwagandha or winter cherry: Said to give the "vitality and sexual energy of a horse," this is one of the Ayurvedic herbs that is hitting the fitness world "big time." Ashwagandha is called an adaptagenic herb, similar to ginseng in traditional Chinese medicine, which means that it supports the adrenal glands rather than taxing them further, as would caffeine, and so helps to increase immunity, or *ojas*. In addition, it has been shown to have a specific affinity for the male reproductive system. It increases Kapha, which makes it helpful to bodybuilders who want to add strength and muscle tissue, but it can also increase *ama,* or a toxic buildup in the system, if used improperly or in excess. It should be blended with digestive herbs to balance Kapha. Adding ashwagandha to warm milk, honey, and a pinch of long pepper will enhance digestion and help to decrease the Kapha effects. This is just one example of why it is important to consult a qualified practitioner when working with medicinal herbs and supplements.

Gotu kola or brahmi: This is one of the most beloved Ayurvedic herbs and one of my favorites. It balances all three constitutional types and is rejuvenative for almost all the tissues in the body. Its most specific use is for the nervous system and the brain. It offers calm, mental clarity, and focus and at the same time can help to decrease excess body fat.

Goksur or Tribilus terrestris: With balancing properties for all three constitutional types, this herb can help to strengthen and flush the kidneys, increasing the "life force." (In traditional Chinese medicine, weak kidneys are considered a sign of depleted life force.) It can also rejuvenate the liver and other Pitta organs and can help to calm and balance the Vata nervous system. Blended with ashwagandha, it can strengthen the reproductive system and increase sperm production, which is explained as increased *ojas,* or life force or strength. This is why it is frequently used by bodybuilders.

Guggulu: This is another Ayurvedic herb or resin that is becoming popular in the mainstream and fitness worlds. It has balancing effects on the body that can actually help to restore homeostasis. It can help to lower cholesterol levels that are too high but seems not to lower them past the point of normal for any particular individual. In addition, it helps to reduce fat and remove toxins, and it goes deep into the tissue to cleanse and rejuvenate.

Gymnema sylvestre: This is called the "sugar killer." It actually reduces cravings for the sweet taste. Yet one more Ayurvedic herb that is becoming popular in the fitness world, *Gymnema sylvestre* can help to balance blood sugar levels. It has been shown to help the beta cells of the pancreas produce insulin more efficiently, which in turn makes sugar metabolism more efficient and reduces insulin resistance. This is one of the herbs included in Be Trim tea.

Shatavari: The name of this herb translates to "she who has one hundred husbands." It is a tonic and rejuvenating herb for the female reproductive system, helping to balance menstrual problems and increase fertility. It is cooling and clarifying to the mind and body and helps nourish the tissues and purify the bloodstream.

Triphala: This herb is a potent antioxidant and yet is gently formulated to support the body's natural cleansing process. Not a laxative, triphala actually has toning qualities that help the colon contract on its own. It also helps to remove mucus from the intestinal tract and can assist in balancing all three constitutional types. It is made up of three different fruits: amla or amalaki, which is rejuvenative for Pitta and the plant source that is highest in vitamin C in the world; haritaki, which helps with either diarrhea or constipation by regulating the colon and balances Vata; and bibhitaki, which is rejuvenative for Kapha and helps to cleanse excess mucus from the colon and tone the bowel.

Other herbs used both in Ayurvedic medicinal formulas and in cooking, such as sandalwood, saffron, and lotus, are wonderful for calming the nerves and clarifying the mind, but to mention them all would be well beyond the scope or purpose of this book. If you'd like to know more about them, please see pages 306 and 317.

Protein Powders

Real food is always best, but if you're in a hurry and don't have time to eat, a protein shake is certainly better than not eating at all. I also recommend protein shakes for postworkout refueling. Too many people train hard and then run around doing errands without ever having stopped to eat. This is actually detrimental to your training and your health, because after a workout, your cells are waiting for replenishment. Combining a whey protein with 2 ounces of juice or almond milk or skim milk and 4 to 6 ounces of water, then mixing in some fresh berries or cardamom or cocoa, is a great way to refuel the body with simple carbohydrates, which *are* helpful after a workout. Adding them to the protein powder after a workout is the best way to use them, because they will help move the amino acids from the protein powder into the cells more quickly to be used for growth and repair. This is the one time you want to increase insulin.

For best digestion, I usually recommend that people rotate their protein powders. Whey protein will be the most efficient for moving amino acids into the cells, but an excess of concentrated dairy products like whey protein can increase mucus and congestion in some people, so pay attention to how you feel. The same holds true for soy protein: it can be difficult for some people to absorb and digest, so try to use it no more than once or twice a week. Organic rice protein is not as biologically beneficial as whey protein because it doesn't contain all the essential amino acids, but if it's mixed with almond milk, it becomes a complete protein, and if it's the only one you digest well, it will serve the purpose.

Whey protein powder: Look for a product from a reputable company so that you can be sure it contains a good-quality whey formula with a highly efficient blend of ion exchanged, microfiltered, and hydrolyzed whey sources that will provide the best absorption and the highest level of amino acids. Seek out products that are manufactured from cows *not* treated with BGH (bovine growth hormone) and that contain no artificial sweeteners. A good formula may also contain branched chain amino acids and L-glutamine. I personally recommend Solgar's whey, which is an excellent whey protein and a very clean product.

Soy protein powder: Look for a product from a good company that contains a concentrated amount of high-quality soy protein, saponins, and the isoflavones genistein and daidzein. Use this in rotation with other protein powders, not more than twice a week, unless otherwise instructed by your health care practitioner.

Metagenics Ultra Clear: This is an organic brown rice–based protein powder/medical food that is designed for use during cleansing but can also be used as a protein supplement. It is easily digestible and hypoallergenic. It contains no gluten, corn, yeast, soy, dairy, artificial coloring or flavoring, and no animal products. It specifically contains amino acids and nutrients, including L-glutathione, L-cysteine, N-acetylcysteine, taurine, green tea catechins, and others, to assist the liver's ability to function.

This product can be purchased only through a medical practitioner such as a doctor, a nutritionist, a chiropractor, or a naturopathic physician. You can also contact the company (see page 306) or log on to our Web site at www.thebalancedapproach.com for more details. Alternatively, you can use any organic rice protein, which can be found in health food stores but will not be as beneficial as Ultra Clear due to the lack of nutrients.

Sports Nutrition Supplements

Electrolyte replacement: These are specialized rehydration formulas providing a unique blend of minerals found in the muscle cells. They should include a combination of sodium, potassium, magnesium, sulfur, and simple carbohydrates in the form of glucose polymers to delay the onset of fatigue from sweating during strenuous activity.

While many people seem to be as frightened of salt as they are of fat, anyone who trains for more than an hour to an hour and a half, especially at a high altitude or in a very dry climate, *needs* to increase his or her salt intake. Regular table salt has most of the trace minerals removed and will increase water retention. Celtic sea salt, sea salt, and orsa salt still have trace minerals intact and will help to balance your electrolytes. Potassium from vegetable broths and proper sodium replacement are critical to recovery and performance.

If you feel lethargic, bloated, or unusually tired after you exercise, you may have an electrolyte imbalance. Try adding ¼ teaspoon of sea salt to your soups, or eat a few good-quality chips without hydrogenated fats and preservatives, such as Kettle Chips or Terra Chips—these will be good carbohydrate replacements that contain no wheat or gluten and have good sea salt. People with low blood pressure, and Vatas, especially need more salt, particularly if they live in a cool, dry climate. People who live by the ocean may not have this problem.

You can make your own electrolyte replacement formula by adding ⅛ to ½ teaspoon of sea salt to an 8-ounce glass of lemonade or limeade. One of my personal favorites is Summertime Lime Quencher by Odwalla; it's an all-natural limeade with water and agave sugar. Not only does it make a perfect electrolyte replacement, but it's also a wonderfully cooling and soothing Pitta drink. With the sea salt added it's the perfect drink to take on a long hike.

L-Glutamine: Produced by the liver, this is the most abundant amino acid in the body. It has been shown to support the building and maintenance of lean muscle tissue and has been used in hospital settings to promote overall health and repair the intestinal tract. The use of glutamine has been correlated with increased fat metabolism and improved mental clarity. It is used by the brain to manufacture neurotransmitters. And since we have the same neurotransmitters in the brain as in the colon, it makes sense that improving colon function will also increase brain function by helping the body to deal with mental and physical stress. In addition, glutamine has also been shown to alleviate blood sugar problems by decreasing insulin resistance. Olympic strength coach Charles Poliquin uses it to help his athletes accelerate muscle glycogen resynthesis after exercise without elevating insulin levels, thus helping them to lose body fat.

CLA: Conjugated linolenic acid (CLA) is a naturally occurring fatty acid that may support healthy glucose and insulin metabolism as well as help to increase lean body mass and decrease body fat, particularly for people with elevated stress-related cortisol levels. Stress and increased cortisol have been shown to increase abdominal fat in certain individuals.

Branched chain amino acids: These include valine, leucine, and isoleucine. These supplements are expensive but can be beneficial for athletes (especially non–meat eaters) and those who train strenu-ously, because branched chain amino acids are the first to be depleted during training and may therefore need to be replenished in order to maximize protein synthesis and minimize protein breakdown.

Cleansing Products

Aloe vera: Taken from the aloe plant, this product can help to regulate sugar and fat metabolism and improve digestion in all three constitu-tional types. A tonic for the liver and spleen, it cools Pitta and lowers Kapha at the same time, which is why I recommend a Green Drink (page 172) three to five times a week for Pittas who are trying to cool down and Kaphas who are trying to lose weight. In excess, how-ever, it can be too cooling for Vatas. It is also mildly laxative, anti-inflammatory, and soothing for the female reproductive system. It can promote menstruation and should not be taken during pregnancy.

Liquid chlorophyll: Taken from the green pigment in plants, chloro-phyll is very similar in chemical structure to human hemoglobin. The difference is that where hemoglobin contains iron, chlorophyll con-tains magnesium. One of the reasons people drink wheat grass, alfalfa, barley, or spirulina is that these plants contain very high con-centrations of chlorophyll and can help to "purify" or cleanse toxins from the bloodstream. Do you remember the chlorophyll gum that was recommended to improve bad breath? Bad breath is usually a sign of a toxic colon, and chlorophyll helps to remove the toxins. It is also a good source of magnesium, a mineral in which many people are deficient.

Milk thistle/silymarin: This is one of the most potent liver-protecting Western herbs known to man. Milk thistle contains an active com-pound called silymarin that has been shown to protect the liver against alcohol abuse and hepatitis and against free-radical damage. It stimulates the production of new liver cells and can also help to re-juvenate the kidneys, adrenals, and bowel.

Red Clover Supreme: I personally like this formula very much. It is a liver-cleansing formula in liquid tincture form that is made by Gaia Herbs and is available in most health food stores. It is a blood and lymphatic alterative formula, which means that it can aid in the metabolism and elimination of toxins from the tissues. It can also help to cool excess heat in the blood and the liver.

Scudders Supreme: This is a lymph-cleansing formula in liquid tincture form that acts to replace catabolic tissue with new, healthy, more vibrant tissue.

Triphala: See page 183.

Essential Fatty Acids

These are the good guys! They help to lower body fat, cholesterol, and triglycerides, and they regulate blood sugar problems and cravings.

EPA/DHA: These are the omega-3 essential fatty acids found in fatty cold-water fish like salmon, mackerel, herring, and sardines. They can also be found in smaller amounts in dark green vegetables such as mustard greens and spinach, as well as in wheat germ oil and canola oil. Essential fatty acids support healthy cholesterol levels, the nervous system, and mental acuity. They can balance hormone levels and help to lower body fat. Our bodies do not manufacture essential fatty acids, so they must be acquired from dietary sources or from supplements in the form of capsules.

Flaxseed oil: For those who are allergic to or do not eat fish, 1 tablespoon of flaxseed oil can provide about 8 grams of omega-3 fatty acids (1 teaspoon is approximately 2.5 grams) in the form of alphalinolenic acid, which the body then converts to EPA/DHA. It provides a vegetarian alternative to fish oils but may take longer to metabolize in some individuals because of the additional enzymatic steps needed to process it into EPA/DHA.

Vegetarian essential fatty acid formulas: These provide EFAs in a blend of flaxseed, evening primrose, borage oil, and lecithin, and others combined with antioxidants to protect freshness. Total EFAs from Health from the Sun (one of my favorites), Udo's Blend of EFAs, or Spectrum Max EPA are all good vegetarian sources.

Hemp seed: This (one of my favorites) is a high-quality protein source that also contains essential fatty acids in the form of alpha-linolenic acid (LNA, omega-3), and gamma-linolenic acid (GLA, omega-6). It has a favorable ratio of omega-3 to omega-6, and since most Americans actually have been consuming *too much* omega-6 in the form of polyunsaturated corn or safflower oil, it is a good alternative. Look for hemp tahini, hemp seed nutter-butter (which has a nice taste), or even hemp ice cream in your health food store. Hemp seed can even replace soy as a source of protein. Caucasians might find it easier to digest, and it's a better environmental product because it requires fewer pesticides and is a more easily rotated crop.

Probiotics

Lactobacillus acidophilus *and* **Bifidobacterium infantis:** These are two of the many kinds of friendly bacteria that help support a balanced intestinal environment. The human intestinal tract hosts hundreds of different species of bacteria. Poor diet, international travel, bad water, and even too many antibiotics are all ways to introduce "bad" bacteria into the intestine. Reinoculating the colon with a good-quality probiotic formula can help to put the digestive system back on track. Be sure to get yours from a reputable company, refrigerated, in a health food store, and not more than three to six weeks old. I usually recommend Metagenics Dairy Free Ultra Flora. New Chapter, PB8, Jarrow, and Natural Factors are also good brands that you can find in health food stores and that have good combinations of bacteria. Many of my clients have seen substantial improvement in digestion simply by eliminating irritating foods from their diet and adding probiotics, EFAs, and glutamine for a period of time.

Adrenal Supportive Herbs

These are "tonic" herbs called adaptagens, which means that they help the body, nervous system, and adrenal glands to handle stress. They support the system without overstimulation. Taken over a period of two to three weeks, a good adrenal support formula usually helps people feel stronger, more grounded, and clear minded, with more balanced energy—and they don't aggravate the nervous system as caffeine would do. They support it. Using adaptagens can actually help you wean off caffeine by supporting the adrenals. Once you feel stronger and less fatigued, you just don't need as much caffeine to keep going or to push on.

Ashwagandha: See page 182.

Astragalus: Popular as a Chinese tonic herb that protects and supports the immune system, astragalus also helps the adrenal glands deal with stress, increasing overall stamina during extreme physical activity. In addition, it can promote digestion and metabolism and, overall, it helps a weakened body regain strength.

Gingko biloba: This traditional Chinese herb has been shown to help increase circulation, thereby elevating brain function and clarity. It has been helpful in decreasing the negative side effects of dementia and Alzheimer's disease and may play a role in protecting against declining intellectual function owing to its ability to increase neurotransmitter function and blood flow to the cells. Ginko has also been shown to decrease platelet aggregation or clumping, oxidative stress, and free-radical damage to cell tissue.

Gotu kola or brahmi: See page 182.

Siberian ginseng: This is from a different botanical family than American, Korean, or Chinese ginseng, all of which are more stimulating. Siberian ginseng is called an adaptagenic herb because it can help to strengthen and support the adrenal glands and reproductive organs. It has also been shown to enhance the immune system, increase circulation, and help manage stress. It can offer overall strength to the body.

Shatavari: See page 183.

Gingko gotu kola: This is a product I love. Made by Frontier Herbs and Rosemary Gladstar—one of the most-beloved and skilled herbalists in the country—it blends many of the adrenal-supportive herbs mentioned above.

Vitamins

I usually recommend a daily multivitamin with additional antioxidants. Non–meat eaters should look for a vegetarian support formula because they need additional B_{12} and folic acid, and women need a formula with additional iron and folic acid. Vitamin B_6, vitamin B_{12}, and folic acid have also been shown to lower homocysteine levels (elevated homocysteine is an indicator of heart disease).

There are three kinds of vitamins available in most health food stores. Although they are usually a bit more expensive, I would recommend that you look for "food-grown" supplements from New Chapter or Mega Foods, which are available in most health food stores and are actually all food. We are able to absorb these more easily than those that are synthetically formulated, since the body knows what to do with food and herbs. Solgar and Country Life are reputable manufacturers of synthetic formulas, and Rainbow or Super Nutrition makes food-blended vitamins—that is, a formula made up of synthetics blended with herbs and natural food substances.

Minerals

Almost 40 percent of Americans have been shown to be magnesium deficient. A good mineral supplement containing additional herbs and minerals like horsetail, silica, and hydroxyapatite has been shown to increase bone density. Take your minerals in the evening, either with your evening meal or in a warm drink before bed. Magnesium is a muscle relaxant that can help you sleep. Look for those from the companies listed above, or ask your local health food store for a recommendation.

A Program of Supplements for the Average Person

Most herbs and supplements should be taken five to six days a week, with one or two days' rest, unless otherwise specified by your practitioner or health care provider. Make sure you check with a health care provider before taking *any* medications.

This day is organized so that you get up early and do your workout in the morning. If you are a night person or work other than from nine to five, make sure you still take your L-glutamine in the morning and evening and your vitamins and EFAs with meals. Use the protein shake after your workout, whether it's in the morning or the evening, and take the adrenal support herbs at midmorning and midafternoon.

When you wake up: Approximately 5 grams of L-glutamine powder dissolved in 2 ounces of warm water, taken on an empty stomach. The higher your level of stress, the more you ought to use. Studies have shown no negative side effects from dosages up to 25 to 40 grams per day.

Glutamine is good for mobilizing fat, maintaining lean muscle tissue, healing the colon, and helping the body deal with stress.

Wait 10 minutes, then have a Green Drink (particularly good for Pitta and Kapha) 3 to 5 times a week:

   1 tablespoon aloe vera juice (Naturade Detox Formula is one of
      my favorites)
   1 tablespoon liquid chlorophyll
   2 to 3 ounces organic cranberry juice

If you are really toxic or trying to cleanse the liver, you may also want to add some additional milk thistle extract or Red Clover Supreme from Gaia Herbs—2 droppers for a period of 2 weeks.

Eat ½ a piece of fruit or a small portion of protein, if necessary, to get you going.

Work out, walk, etc.

Have your postworkout protein shake.

With breakfast: A good-quality multivitamin from a reputable company such as New Chapter, Country Life, or Solgar (see page 191 for further options). This should be taken with food for maximum absorption.

Take 1 tablespoon liquid flaxseed oil or flax-blended oil. (I usually recommend flax rather than fish oil because some people just can't tolerate fish oil in the morning. If you don't have a problem, you can alternate flaxseed oil with fish oil.)

Good fats are necessary in the morning for balancing hormonal responses and avoiding the insulin spikes from sugar and simple carbohydrates that would lead to blood sugar swings. Some people add them to their cottage cheese. Just don't cook them, they are not meant to be heated.

Midmorning: Depending on your stress level, take adrenal support (page 189). (This is particularly helpful to people who are trying to reduce their caffeine intake. Using adrenal support is a kinder, gentler—and therefore more helpful—way to cut caffeine than simply going cold turkey. These supplments help build balanced energy; they are not stimulants. As the adrenals and nervous system become stronger, there is less need for caffeine to get going.) For best absorption, these herbs should not be taken with food. The amount is usually determined by weight or constitutional type, and recommended amounts are listed on the label. Vatas and Pittas need more adrenal support, but usually a smaller actual quantity than heavier Kaphas.

With lunch: Take another multivitamin if your program is for "2 a day." If you're taking "1 a day," take it with breakfast.
Take 1 to 2 EPA/DHA fish oil capsules before your meal to avoid "tasting" them as you might if you took them after eating a meal.

Midafternoon: Take a second dose of adrenal support.

With afternoon snack: Depending on your weight and your need to decrease Kapha, take 1 to 2 EPA/DHA capsules.

Dinner: Take a multimineral either at dinner or at bedtime.
Mineral formulas with magnesium usually help people to relax and fall asleep because magnesium is a muscle relaxant.

Before bed, on an empty stomach: Take 5 grams of L-glutamine in 2 ounces of warm water to mobilize fat and maintain lean muscle tissue or for high physical or emotional stress.

If you have digestive problems: I would also recommend adding a probiotic to the formula. If they are not enteric-coated to avoid their being broken down by stomach acid, it is usually recommended that you try to take them approximately 30 minutes after a meal, when your stomach acids are not so strong. If you eat dairy, you can open a capsule and put it in your yogurt or cottage cheese, or even into a protein shake *after* it has been blended.

If needed, you can also take milk thistle (follow the directions on the label for dosages) or a blended liver-cleansing supplement such as Gaia's Red Clover Supreme before bed.

Again, I must emphasize that the above are only simple and basic recommendations, that they should not be interpreted as medical advice, and that you should seek out a qualified herbalist or nutritionist to help determine the specific program that would be right for you.

CHAPTER TEN

Recipes for Staying in Balance with Herbs and Spices

Now that you understand the principles of eating to keep your body and mind in balance and have done your gentle cleanse, it's time to get started. Changing your way of eating can seem a bit overwhelming at first, but it's really a lot easier than you think.

First, I'm going to give you some basic guidelines that can be adapted to create an endless number of delicious, quick, wholesome, and nutritious meals for yourself and your entire family. Please remember that just five years ago, I myself didn't know much about this approach to eating and good health. Coming from New York, where I (and, it seemed to me, everyone else) ate out all the time, I was starting from scratch, didn't cook, and was as confused and frustrated about what to eat as so many of you. So I understand how you might be feeling, and you can be assured that if I could do it, you can, too.

As we've already discussed, cooking with the fresh, whole foods, herbs, and spices you now have on hand is really much easier, and faster, than cooking with the bland, overprocessed, carbohydrate-laden foods you've probably been used to eating. The fresher your basic ingredients, the closer they are to their natural state, the more flavor they will have on their own, and, consequently, the less you'll have to do to them to make them taste really great. In fact, using just a few ingredients and cooking them simply to retain their natural flavors, you can prepare wonderful meals in less than thirty minutes.

Working with Gigia Kolouch, the talented and inspiring food historian and cooking school teacher who has contributed many of the recipes and information in this chapter, has helped me to overcome my fear of cooking. I've learned from Gigia why Mediterranean, Asian, and other cuisines that we think of as "ethnic" seem so much simpler, cleaner, and more flavorful than what has come to be considered the more common American diet. Indira Gupta and Amadea Morningstar have been inspirational and helped to teach me about traditional Indian and Ayurvedic cooking techniques.

CONTINENTAL- VERSUS ETHNIC-STYLE COOKING

The foods Americans most often eat now are still those that were brought over by the early settlers from Germany and the United Kingdom, and the techniques used to cook those foods are mainly what we call "continental style." These techniques were invented in France and Italy during the Middle Ages and are based primarily on chemical reactions, which means that measuring and careful watching are essential to the outcome. For example, if you are making a classic white sauce, you must carefully measure the butter, flour, and liquid and make sure they are blended and heated properly to ensure a sauce of the right consistency and taste.

The cooking methods used prior to the introduction of continental cuisine—going as far back as the ancient Greeks and Romans—were much simpler. They didn't rely on chemical reactions, and they didn't use so many dairy products or as much fat to create richness and satisfaction. In consequence, they were much more dependent on the use of all six flavors to make their food taste good. That is the method of cooking we're going to be discussing here. It's the cooking style used in most ethnic or "peasant" cuisines, which rely on simple ingredients and lots of spices and flavorings to enhance nutritional value, improve digestion, and satisfy taste. It's a much more liberating way to cook because it frees you to experiment with flavor combinations that appeal particularly to you; it's easier, because it isn't so dependent on mastering technique; and it gives you the pleasure of tasting fresh, clean flavors that are incredibly delicious and, at the same time, contribute to your digestive health.

EXPERIMENTING WITH HERBS AND SPICES

If you are learning about herbs and spices for the first time, it would probably be a good idea to start by buying a few—perhaps eight or ten—that you think you might enjoy and would like to learn more about. Look at the list on page 24 to get an idea of those I generally recommend that clients try first. If you go to a greengrocer that sells fresh herbs, or to a health food or other store that sells dried herbs and spices in bulk, you'll be able to smell before you buy. Undoubtedly there will be aromas that particularly appeal to you and others that don't. Let your nose be your guide and, most likely, you won't be disappointed.

The following lists were put together by Gigia to help my clients understand some of the most traditional flavor combinations for a variety of ethnic cuisines. See which of them sound good to you or which ones you might have tried and enjoyed in a restaurant. If you like Indian or Italian or Mexican food, give those combinations a try. And remember, the dishes you create don't have to conform to anyone else's idea of what the food "should" taste like; it only has to taste good *to you*.

Mediterranean Flavor Combinations

Italian/French

Rosemary/thyme/red wine
Sorrel, watercress, or chervil/lemon or white wine
Thyme/lemon/pepper
Olives/sun-dried tomatoes/garlic/rosemary
White wine/garlic/parsley/tomatoes (optional)
Olive oil/garlic/basil
Anchovies/capers/lemon or white wine/garlic/parsley/tomatoes
    (optional)
Sage/pasta or meat/nuts/Parmesan cheese

Basil/oregano/thyme/bay leaf/rosemary
Butter/shallots/thyme or tarragon/white wine

Italy and France use wine and vinegar for cooking.

Middle Eastern

Turmeric/coriander/cumin/ginger/cinnamon
Lemon/olives or olive oil/garlic/parsley or mint
Tomatoes/garlic/olive oil/cinnamon/allspice
Garlic/olive oil/tomatoes/basil

*Greece and the Middle East use lemon and chicken stock
for cooking.*

All of the Mediterranean flavor combinations occur in soups, sauces, pestos, stews, pastas, grains, and meat or poultry or fish dishes.

Asian Flavor Combinations

Japanese

Sesame oil/soy sauce/sugar/mirin (You can use maple syrup or
Sucanat in place of processed sugar.)
Lemon/miso/soy sauce or rice wine vinegar
Mirin/soy sauce
Ginger/soy sauce/sugar/sesame oil
Wasabi/ginger/soy sauce/citrus

Thai/Vietnamese

Lemongrass/lime/ginger or laos/cilantro/fish sauce
Peanuts/tamarind/lemon or lime/fish sauce/sugar
Coconut milk/lime/fish sauce/basil or mint
Rice vinegar/fish sauce/chilies/lemon, lime, or tamarind/
sugar/garlic

Chinese

Fermented black beans/garlic/ginger
Soy sauce/cornstarch/Chinese cooking wine/sugar/chili/
garlic paste (optional)
Soy sauce/rice wine vinegar/chili oil/ginger (optional)

Indian

Yogurt, lemon or lime/ginger/garlic/chilies/garam masala
Ginger/garlic/garam masala/tomatoes/coconut milk
Tamarind/chilies/ginger/curry powder
Mustard seeds/fennel seeds/cumin seeds/ginger/garlic
Cumin/coriander/cardamom/turmeric

COOKING FROM THE MEDITERRANEAN PANTRY

Mediterranean cuisine is probably the most familiar to Americans and the one whose flavors are most similar to our own. Not only is it easy to cook at home, it's also readily accessible almost everywhere in the country when you're eating out: a soup to start, followed by fish with vegetables sautéed in oil and garlic, a salad, and a small sweet, and you've got a delicious, healthy meal for Vata, Pitta, or Kapha.

Americans tend to think of Italian food as being based on pasta and cheese, but that's not how Italians eat at home in Italy. (In fact, for whatever reason, many healthy indigenous cuisines seem to become heavier and more starch-laden the minute they hit American soil.) Actually, Italian home cooking, based on the Mediterranean food pyramid, is acknowledged by nutritionists and health professionals to be among the healthiest in the world.

COOKING FROM THE LATIN AMERICAN PANTRY

Mexican is another popular cuisine that has suffered an undeservedly bad reputation for being fatty, starchy, and generally unhealthy. In fact, at a continuing education weight-loss class I attended recently, one speaker offered the sweeping generalization that all ethnic cuisines are much too high in fat. Actually, however, indigenous Mexican cuisine is based mainly on combining vegetarian ingredients—such as black beans, anasazi, pinto, or navy beans combined with grains like corn, rice, and, to a lesser degree, wheat—to create complete proteins. It can be easily adapted to include lean animal proteins such as chicken, fish, or lean beef. Mexican cooking doesn't use very many spices. Cumin, oregano, thyme, cinnamon, and all-

The Traditional Healthy Mediterranean Diet Pyramid

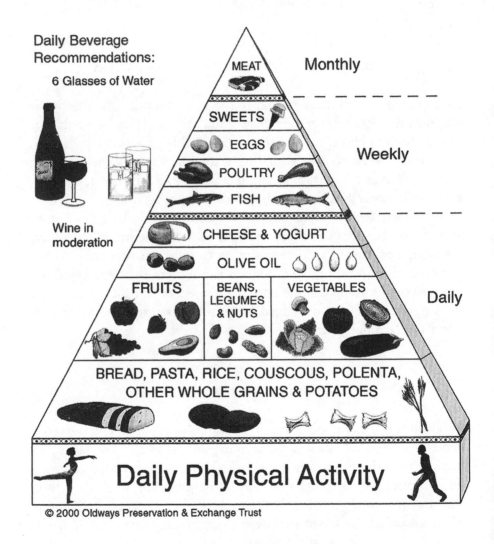

Daily Beverage Recommendations:

6 Glasses of Water

Wine in moderation

Monthly

MEAT

SWEETS

Weekly

EGGS

POULTRY

FISH

CHEESE & YOGURT

OLIVE OIL

FRUITS   BEANS, LEGUMES & NUTS   VEGETABLES

Daily

BREAD, PASTA, RICE, COUSCOUS, POLENTA, OTHER WHOLE GRAINS & POTATOES

Daily Physical Activity

The Traditional Healthy
Latin American Diet Pyramid

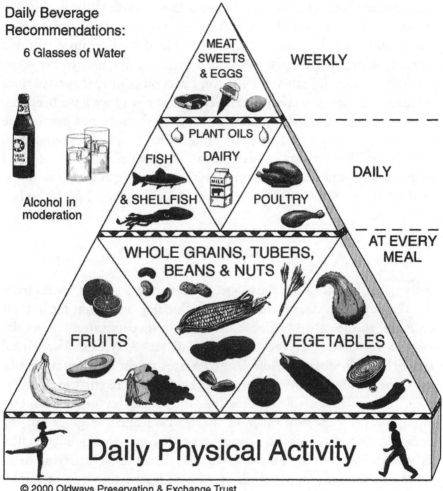

Daily Beverage Recommendations:

6 Glasses of Water

Alcohol in moderation

MEAT SWEETS & EGGS

WEEKLY

PLANT OILS

FISH & SHELLFISH

DAIRY

POULTRY

DAILY

WHOLE GRAINS, TUBERS, BEANS & NUTS

AT EVERY MEAL

FRUITS

VEGETABLES

Daily Physical Activity

spice are among the most popular (and now you know that they also help to enhance digestion and cut body fat). But it does use a variety of condiments like salsas, picante sauces, and guacamole for added flavor, and those can be either bought or created without adding very much work on the part of the cook.

And, like Mediterranean food, this kind of cooking is readily available in restaurants throughout the country. A fajita, for example, can be made with rice and beans and also with shrimp, chicken, or beef. It will also usually include sautéed onions and peppers. Add some guacamole if you're a Pitta, and a bit of sour cream if you're a Vata, or some salsa to raise the Kapha digestive fire, and you're set to go. When I visited Peru and Ecuador, I was pleasantly surprised once again to see that they traditionally eat just the way we have been discussing. They have light breakfasts with fresh fruit and homemade yogurt, cheese, and coffee. Their larger meal is served around 2:30 P.M. It usually consists of fish, meat, vegetables, and/or rice and beans. South Americans do not use much wheat—quinoa is the staple grain in Peru and the Andes, and is considered the food of the gods.

COOKING FROM THE ASIAN PANTRY

Moving halfway around the globe, we can take a similar lesson from the Asian pantry. Asians don't use much dairy or animal fat in their cooking, so the entire cuisine is designed to incorporate as many flavors as possible to replace the flavor of fat. A typical Asian meal served in a restaurant in the United States might be a small cup of miso soup followed by salmon teriyaki, some rice, stir-fried vegetables, and a salad with ginger dressing. Spices and flavorings would include not only the soy sauce in the teriyaki and the ginger in the dressing, but also wasabi. A meal like this includes good, healthy protein, it incorporates all six tastes, and it would be satisfying to all three constitutional types while still being light enough for a Kapha or anyone trying to lose weight, and sweet enough (from the rice, ginger, and soy sauce) to soothe either a Vata or Pitta imbalance. The wasabi and ginger are great for reducing body fat and Kapha.

The Traditional Healthy
Asian Diet Pyramid

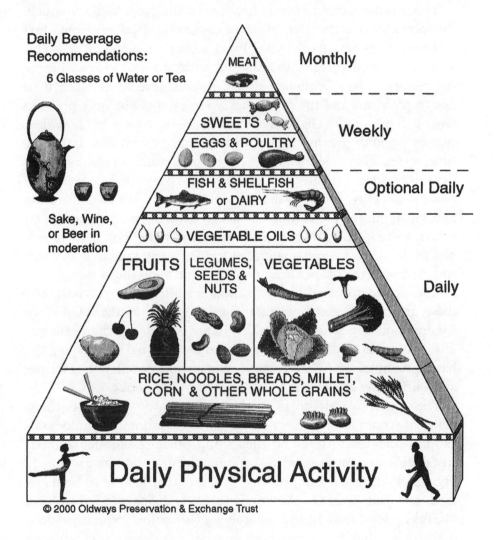

Daily Beverage
Recommendations:

6 Glasses of Water or Tea

Sake, Wine,
or Beer in
moderation

MEAT · Monthly

SWEETS · Weekly
EGGS & POULTRY

FISH & SHELLFISH
or DAIRY · Optional Daily

VEGETABLE OILS

FRUITS · LEGUMES, SEEDS & NUTS · VEGETABLES · Daily

RICE, NOODLES, BREADS, MILLET, CORN & OTHER WHOLE GRAINS

Daily Physical Activity

ABOUT THE RECIPES

The recipes that follow come from four different contributors, all of whom are devoted to the concept of getting our food from clean, sustainable, mostly organic, free-range, environmentally friendly, and humanely raised sources.

The first and largest group of recipes comes from Gigia Kolouch, the food historian and Denver-based cooking instructor whom I first met four years ago. At the time, I was seeing more and more clients with severe food allergies and candida problems who kept asking me for recipes. I was beginning to see the connection between their health problems and the foods they were eating. The only problem was, I didn't cook! Gigia saved my neck—not only by providing recipes I could give my clients with dietary restrictions, but, over time, by teaching me how to make her wonderfully simple and unbelievably delicious dishes for myself. Her cooking has incredible *prana,* or energy, and she's made it not only easy but also nurturing and satisfying for me and my clients to experiment with herbs and spices in the kitchen. She's helped me to apply the Ayurvedic principles of the six tastes and qualities of food to every kind of ethnic cuisine, and with the recipes here, you'll be able to do the same.

The second group of recipes is more traditionally Ayurvedic, and these are contributed by Indira Gupta, owner of the Madrid to Madras Cooking School in Boulder. Indira is skilled in the use of traditional Indian and Ayurvedic spices and dedicated to teaching the basic principles of Ayurveda to a mainstream population. Her joy and spirit bring energy and life to everything she cooks.

The "guest contributors" to this chapter are world-class chefs, many of whom are members of the Chefs Collaborative, an organization dedicated to teaching clients and other restaurateurs about sustainable agriculture and to cooking clean, good-quality, mostly organic food, raised and provided in a way that is kind to both our land and our animals. All of these chefs manage to transform "healthy" food into an incomparable gastronomic experience on a daily basis. All of them have been unbelievably generous in allowing me to include their recipes here. I am truly honored to be able to share them with you. I felt very strongly about including these amazing "food artists" in this book to let you know about their dedication to supporting local organic farmers and their commitment to developing a sense of community and humanity with their food suppliers. Many of them work extremely long hours and still find time to shop at local organic farmers' markets for superior-quality food items. Sustainable agriculture is an important issue for these chefs.

Finally, there are my own "quick and easy" shortcuts (taking literally twenty-five minutes or less) for using high-quality prepared foods to make nourishing and tasty meals. When I started to incorporate Ayurvedic principles into my life, this was the only way I knew how to do it, and I still cook this way much of the time, simply because I run a business and don't generally have as much time as I would like to dedicate to cooking. These shortcuts are a way to insure that I always have access to good-quality food even with limited time, and you, too, can use them to make sure the food you eat is nurturing and delicious, even when you don't have time to cook.

THE RECIPES

All of these recipes are designed to work for all three constitutional types. In any instance where this is not the case, it will be so noted in the recipe.

The nutritional breakdowns have been calculated and provided by Gigia Kolouch.

Soups

Soups are warming, nurturing, and a wonderful way to start your meal. They are good for all constitutional types, including Pittas (unless it is in the heat of summer). Remember that warm temperature is not the same thing as hot, meaning spicy, and Pittas would do well to flavor their soups with the sweeter herbs and spices, while Vatas and Kaphas can use those that are "spicier" and more pungent.

From Gigia

MISO SOUP

Miso is a paste made from fermented soybeans, grains, and salt. It cleanses toxins from the body and provides digestive enzymes. Take care not to boil the miso, as boiling will destroy the enzymes. It will stay fresh for months in the refrigerator and can be used to replace salt or salty cheese in a recipe.

Miso comes in a variety of flavors. The lighter colors are suitable for spring and summer, while the darker reds are best in fall and winter.

Makes 6 servings

1 (5-inch) piece kombu sea vegetable	3 tablespoons white miso
2 dried shiitake mushrooms	2 green onions, chopped
6 cups water	Slivered lemon rind

Bring the kombu and mushrooms to a boil in the water, then lower the heat and simmer for 15 minutes. Strain the broth. (This is known as dashi and may be used as the stock base for any light Japanese soup.)

Bring the dashi to a boil, then turn off the heat. In a cup, dissolve the miso in 3 tablespoons of the hot stock and add it to the stock in the pot.

Ladle the miso soup into 6 soup bowls and garnish each serving with the chopped green onion and slivered lemon rind.

Per serving: 37 calories; 1 gram fat; 2 grams protein; 7 grams carbohydrate

Variations: Garnish the soup with thinly sliced mushrooms, chopped greens, seaweed, or grated carrot instead of the green onion and lemon rind.

From Jennifer

QUICK AND EASY BUTTERNUT SQUASH, SWEET POTATO, AND SPINACH SOUP

I'm very proud of this recipe because it was my first. The cumin, coriander, turmeric, and fennel in this soup are cooling for summer and for Pittas. In winter, you might want to use garam masala instead because it's more heating. I like to serve this with sautéed kale as a vegetable and 4 to 6 ounces of marinated tofu or chicken or shrimp as a protein.

Makes 1 serving

½ butternut squash	½ teaspoon cumin
½ garnet yam or sweet potato	½ teaspoon coriander
½ bunch fresh spinach, washed	½ teaspoon turmeric
2 to 3 ounces vanilla almond, rice, soy, skim, or buttermilk	½ teaspoon fennel
2 to 3 ounces vegetable broth	½ teaspoon orsa, sea salt, or celtic salt
4 to 6 ounces water	1 tablespoon maple syrup, for garnish

Bake the squash and yam in a 450-degree oven for 1 hour, or until the flesh is easily pierced with a fork.

Discard the seeds from the squash and peel the yam. Cut the vegetables into coarse chunks and puree them in a blender with the spinach, milk, broth, and water. The puree will be rather thick.

Transfer the pureed vegetable mixture to a saucepot, add the spices and salt, and heat thoroughly. Drizzle the maple syrup over the soup just before serving.

Per serving: 338 calories; 4 grams fat; 10 grams protein; 73 grams carbohydrate

Variation: You can leave out the yam and add more spinach and squash to reduce the carbs, but the soup won't be as sweet.

From Gigia

TOFU NOODLE BOWL

This is actually filling enough to be a complete meal, especially for a lighter dinner. Make it without the noodles as a first course soup, or serve a smaller portion with the noodles.

Make this when you have lots of leftover steamed vegetables so you don't have to spend time slicing all the ingredients. Keep the marinated tofu on hand to use for salads, sandwiches, or as a main course with side dishes.

If you dislike or can't digest tofu, you can substitute shrimp, fish, or chicken.

Makes 6 large servings

For the Soup:

8 cups water	6 snow peas
2 tablespoons Bragg's or wheat-free tamari	½ red bell pepper
	½ carrot
1 tablespoon grated fresh ginger	2 kale leaves
2 teaspoons sesame oil	6 ounces rice sticks or rice noodles

For the Tofu:

1 package firm tofu	3 tablespoons honey
2 tablespoons grated fresh ginger	3 tablespoons soy sauce
2 tablespoons sesame oil	¼ cup sake or vegetable broth
2 tablespoons sesame seeds, crushed	

For the soup base, combine the water, tamari, ginger, and sesame oil in a large saucepan. Bring the liquid to a boil, then cover the pan and keep the mixture warm over low heat. (This is another method of making a quick Asian-style broth that may be used for any light soup.)

Preheat the oven to 400 degrees.

Cut the tofu into three rectangles by slicing through it lengthwise. Cut the rectangles in half, then cut them diagonally into triangles. Place them in a baking pan large enough to hold them in one layer. Combine the ginger, sesame oil, sesame seeds, honey, soy sauce, and sake and pour the marinade mixture over the tofu. Bake in the pre-heated oven for 15 minutes, then remove the pan, turn over the tofu, and return to the oven to bake another 5 minutes, or until all the liquid is evaporated.

(To do this on top of the stove, put 1 teaspoon of sesame oil in a nonstick pan, add the tofu, and, when it begins to color, pour the marinade over it and continue cooking until it turns dark brown.)

While the tofu is baking, cut the snow peas, red pepper, and carrot into very thin strips. Shred the kale leaves into thin ribbons.

Bring the broth back to a boil and add the rice sticks. After 2 minutes, add the vegetables and cook 1 minute longer. Spoon the soup into bowls and place the marinated tofu on top of the rice noodles.

Per serving: 487 calories; 16 grams fat; 22 grams protein; 68 grams carbohydrate

From Gigia

MINESTRA DI VERDURA CON PESTO (Vegetable Soup with Pesto)

This winter or spring soup includes a handy recipe for a vegetarian garlic broth that's quick to make and tastes like a light chicken broth. To speed up the preparation, you can also make the broth with 8 cups of water, ½ cup of white wine, and 3 tablespoons of Bragg's tamari instead of the garlic broth. A nice vegetable soup is a tasty way to add nutritious greens to your diet.

Makes 6 servings

For the Garlic Broth:

2 heads garlic
1 onion
8 cups water
1 bay leaf

2 parsley sprigs
2 thyme sprigs or ¼ teaspoon dried
   thyme
1 to 2 teaspoons salt

For the Soup:

1 pound string beans
1 bunch kale
2 leeks
2 tablespoons olive oil
1 teaspoon salt
1 cup pearl barley

1 bay leaf
2 teaspoons dried rosemary
Salt and pepper, to taste
Freshly grated Parmesan cheese, for
   garnish
Pesto (page 252), for garnish

To make the broth, separate the garlic cloves and smash them lightly with a meat pounder or the back of a skillet. Peel the onion and cut it in quarters. Combine all the ingredients in a stockpot and bring the liquid to a boil. Reduce the heat, cover, and simmer 30 minutes. Strain and, if not finishing the soup immediately, refrigerate for 4 to 5 days or freeze for up to 3 months.

To make the soup, top and tail the string beans and cut them in half. Soak the kale to remove the sand and drain it. Then cut off and discard the tough bottom stems and chop it coarsely. Cut off and discard the roots of the leeks, slit them in half, and wash them under running water. Slice the leeks crosswise into thin crescents.

Sauté the leeks in the olive oil, and when they are soft, add the kale and string beans. Add the garlic broth, 1 teaspoon of salt, the barley, bay leaf, and rosemary, and simmer the soup 1 hour, or until the barley and vegetables are cooked through.

Adjust the seasoning with salt and pepper to taste, ladle the soup into individual bowls, and garnish each serving with a sprinkling of grated Parmesan and a dollop of pesto. You can leave out the barley to decrease the carbs.

Per serving (including pesto and cheese): 192 calories; 5 grams fat; 6 grams protein; 32 grams carbohydrate

From Jennifer

QUICK AND EASY CURRIED VEGETABLE SOUP

Makes 2 servings

1 can Health Valley (or any other organic) soup of your choice (black bean, chicken and rice, vegetable, etc.)

¼ package frozen mixed vegetables

¼ to ½ teaspoon curry powder or garam masala, or spices of your choice

3 ounces rice or almond cheese, or Monterey Jack or goat cheese or Cheddar, grated

Combine the soup, vegetables, and spice in a soup pot and heat until the vegetables are defrosted and the soup is piping hot. Spoon into bowls, sprinkle with the grated cheese, and serve.

Per serving: 166 calories; 3 grams fat; 10 grams protein; 25 grams carbohydrate

Vegetables and Salads

Salads, like vegetables, are an important component of every meal. Always remember to dress them with good oils.

From Jennifer

QUICK AND EASY BAKED SQUASH

For a dish that is higher in starch, suitable for Vatas and Pittas, you can use this same preparation to bake a garnet yam or a sweet potato. Squash is sweet and grounding, full of vitamins and fiber, gluten free, low in calories, and lower on the glycemic index than the potato or yam. My own favorite squash is Delicata, which is so sweet that to me it tastes like candy!

Makes 2 servings

1 whole squash (delicata, acorn, dumpling, or butternut)
1 teaspoon ghee
¼ teaspoon cinnamon
⅛ to ¼ teaspoon cardamom
⅛ to ¼ teaspoon nutmeg
Pinch of salt

Preheat the oven to 350 degrees.

Cut the squash in half and scoop out the seeds. Brush the cut side of each half with the ghee and sprinkle with the cinnamon, cardamom, nutmeg, and salt. Place the squash halves cut side up in a baking dish and bake in the preheated oven for 20 to 30 minutes.

The squash is cooked when easily pierced with a fork. Add a drop more ghee and spice if you like before serving.

Per serving: 87 calories; 2 grams fat; 1 gram protein; 17 grams carbohydrate

From Jennifer

QUICK AND EASY SAUTÉED KALE

Use the same preparation for chard, collards, mustard greens, broccoli, or baby bok choy, another sweet favorite of mine that is also high in calcium. Pittas should use the olive oil or ghee; Vatas and Kaphas can use any of the three oils, but Kaphas should try to do with less. Bitter greens combined with mango chutney are great for Pittas and Kaphas because the combination is sweet, astringent, low in calories, and high in fiber and nutrients. This basic dish is great with veggie burgers, omelets, fish, or chicken.

Makes 2 servings

1 tablespoon olive oil, ghee, or sesame oil

1 onion, cut in half and sliced thin

4 to 5 shiitake mushrooms, wiped clean with a damp cloth or paper towel and sliced

½ to 1 red bell pepper, cored, seeded, and sliced

4 stalks kale, or any combination of greens, rinsed and torn

1 tablespoon Patak's mango chutney

Heat the oil of your choice in a pan large enough to hold all the ingredients and sauté the onion until it is golden, soft, and translucent. Add the mushrooms and pepper slices and sauté until the vegetables are soft. Add the kale, cover the pan, and cook 2 to 3 minutes—just long enough to wilt the greens. Transfer the vegetables to a plate, top with the chutney, and serve.

Per serving: 166 calories; 8 grams fat; 4 grams protein; 24 grams carbohydrate

From Gigia

GREEK SALAD

This is a simple version of the colorful and delicious Greek salad. Quick and easy to prepare, it makes a perfect starter or side salad. It's great in the summer for Pittas and Kaphas. Vatas may want to stick with cooked vegetables.

Makes 4 servings

1 bunch Romaine lettuce	½ cup olives
1 cucumber	¼ cup extra virgin olive oil
3 tomatoes	2 tablespoons lemon juice
1 red or green bell pepper	½ teaspoon salt
½ large red onion	Freshly ground black pepper, to taste
½ cup feta cheese, crumbled	½ teaspoon oregano

Wash and dry the lettuce leaves. Chill the lettuce while preparing the rest of the salad. Peel and slice the cucumber. Cut the tomatoes into wedges. Cut the pepper and onion into thin strips. Arrange the lettuce leaves on a plate. Toss the vegetables together and spoon them onto the lettuce. Sprinkle the feta cheese and olives on top. Whisk together the olive oil, lemon juice, salt, pepper, and oregano. Pour the dressing over the salad and serve.

Per serving: 239 calories; 19 grams fat; 6 grams protein; 14 grams carbohydrate

From the Chefs Collaborative: Jesse Cool

ASPARAGUS WITH WARM BALSAMIC DRIZZLE, HERBED CREAM CHEESE, AND RADISHES

Jesse Cool is the proprietor of Flea Street Café and jZcool in Menlo Park, California, and the Cool Café in Stanford, California. For more than twenty-six years, through personal and business endeavors, she has been dedicated to sustainable agriculture and cuisine. Supporting organic farmers, whom she warmly refers to as her heroes and the first real environmental pioneers, she strives to manage her food business so that it reflects her politics and philosophy.

Kaphas may want to substitute goat cheese for the cream cheese in this dish.

Makes 4 to 6 servings

1 pound medium-size asparagus, snapped and stems peeled

1 green onion

1 tablespoon good-quality balsamic vinegar

1 tablespoon tamari or soy sauce

3 tablespoons brown sugar

2 cloves garlic, minced fine

2 tablespoons water

8 ounces softened cream cheese (or substitute fresh goat cheese)

2 tablespoons chopped fresh chives

2 tablespoons chopped fresh tarragon

1 small baguette, sliced 1 inch thick*

Salt and freshly ground pepper

6 radishes, washed and sliced thin

In a steamer basket, over boiling water, steam the asparagus for 3 to 5 minutes, or until tender but not overcooked. Rinse them immediately under cold water and set aside. Cut the top off the onion, trimming away the frayed ends. In a steamer basket, steam the green tops until wilted. Run them under cold water and set aside.

To make the sauce, in a small saucepan, combine the balsamic vinegar, soy sauce, brown sugar, and garlic. Add 2 tablespoons of water. Over medium heat, reduce the liquid by half. Add the reserved green onion and adjust the seasoning.

In a small bowl, combine the cream cheese (or goat cheese), chives, and tarragon.

In a toaster oven or under the broiler, toast one side of each baguette slice. Spread each with a small amount of the cream cheese mixture and season it with salt and pepper. Arrange the radish slices on top of the cream cheese.

Arrange the asparagus on one large platter or 4 to 6 individual salad plates. Drizzle them with the vinaigrette, and arrange the baguette slices near the asparagus. This dish can be served either warm or chilled.

Per serving: 382 calories; 16 grams fat; 12 grams protein; 50 grams carbohydrate

* Jennifer suggests that you might want to try a nongluten substitute for the baguette.

From Gigia

FUL MEDAMES (Fava Bean Salad)

This hearty salad makes use of the Middle Eastern bean ful medames, which is a relative of the fava bean. It's delicious scooped up with pita bread, and it can also be served with a tomato or a whole-grain salad such as tabouli or quinoa for a complete protein source. Canned ful medames can be found in gourmet food shops and in Middle Eastern or Greek markets.

This is an example of how spices can help you to digest the beans. A wonderful dish for Pittas and Kaphas.

Makes 8 servings

1 large onion, coarsely chopped
5 cloves garlic, peeled and minced
⅛ teaspoon cayenne pepper
2 teaspoons ground cumin
1 tablespoon olive oil
3 cups cooked ful medames or fava beans
1 teaspoon salt

1 teaspoon freshly ground black pepper
1 tablespoon extra-virgin olive oil
1 tomato, chopped
½ cup chopped fresh parsley
Juice of 1 lemon
¼ onion, minced

Sauté the chopped onion, 4 cloves of the garlic, the cayenne, and the cumin in the tablespoon of olive oil. Add the beans and cook 10 minutes. Mash some of the beans, then add the remaining garlic and the salt and pepper.

Transfer the bean mixture to a shallow bowl and drizzle it with the extra-virgin olive oil. Top with the chopped tomato, parsley, lemon juice, and minced onion. Serve, if you wish, with pita bread triangles.

Per serving: 75 calories; 4 grams fat; 3 grams protein; 9 grams carbohydrate

Variation: Use any other large, meaty bean, such as cannellini, butter, or garbanzos, in place of the ful medames or fava beans.

From the Chefs Collaborative: Jeffrey Mora

ROASTED ROOT VEGETABLES WITH ARUGULA, WHOLE-GRAIN MUSTARD, AND SHERRY DRESSING

Jeffrey Mora sits on the board of the Earth Communications Office and is the owner of Carnivale restaurant in Monterey, California. Jeff is dedicated to creating a sustainable business. He believes that chefs have a responsibility to provide clean, healthy meals to clients and to educate the public about why sustainable, organic food is important.

Roasting the vegetables makes them sweeter and more digestible. This dish is good for all three constitutional types.

Makes 4 servings

1 celery root, peeled and cut into 8 wedges	3 sprigs thyme
1 pound parsley root, peeled and cut lengthwise	½ cup olive oil
	2 teaspoons sea salt
3 parsnips, peeled and cut 1 inch thick	2 teaspoons coarsely ground black pepper
1 large red onion, cut into large pieces	½ pound arugula
1 head garlic, cloves peeled and left whole	1 recipe sherry dressing (recipe follows)

Preheat the oven to 375 degrees.

Toss together all the ingredients except the arugula and dressing and place them in a roasting pan on the middle shelf of the oven. Roast for 45 minutes to 1 hour, tossing the vegetables every 5 minutes until they are tender. Remove from the oven and cool. When completely cooled, place them in a large bowl, add the arugula and the sherry dressing, and adjust the seasoning if necessary.

Sherry Dressing

1 ounce sherry vinegar	1 tablespoon whole-grain mustard
1 ounce sherry wine	1 shallot, peeled
1 tablespoon honey	1 egg yolk (optional)
1 teaspoon horseradish	6 ounces walnut oil

Place all the ingredients except the oil in a blender. With the motor running, slowly add the oil, blending well after each addition.

Per serving (if you use all the dressing): 651 calories; 50 grams fat; 6 grams protein; 49 grams carbohydrate

From Indira

CUCUMBER RAITA

Here's an example of how Indian cookery uses spices—in this case cumin—to cut the "Kapha" or "mucus" in the yogurt. It's a good dish for Vatas and, in smaller amounts, for Pittas and Kaphas.

Makes 16 servings as a relish

1 large cucumber
2 cups plain yogurt
½ teaspoon salt

½ teaspoon toasted, crushed cumin
   seeds
Pinch of paprika

Wash, peel, and grate the cucumber. Squeeze out all the excess water. Stir in the yogurt to make a smooth mixture. Add the salt and all but a pinch of the cumin and combine. Sprinkle with the reserved cumin and the paprika and serve.

Per serving: 20 calories; 1 gram fat; 1 gram protein; 2 grams carbohydrate

From Gigia

SESAME BROCCOLI SALAD

Makes 8 servings

3 heads broccoli, cut into small
   flowerets (blanched, or slightly
   steamed, if you like)
1 red bell pepper, peeled, seeded, and
   cut in thin strips
1 bunch green onions (white part and 2
   inches of green), sliced thin
1 tablespoon fresh ginger, peeled and
   cut in thin strips

2 tablespoons black sesame seeds,
   toasted in a dry skillet
¼ cup soy sauce
2 tablespoons honey
2 tablespoons canola oil
2 tablespoons sesame oil
¼ cup rice wine vinegar

Toss the vegetables and sesame seeds with the soy sauce, honey, canola oil, sesame oil, and vinegar. Chill before serving. In Ayurveda they would say steaming the vegetables may reduce *prana,* but it will increase digestibility for certain people.

Per serving: 113 calories; 8 grams fat; 2 grams protein; 9 grams carbohydrate

From Chef Peter Berley

SPICY ROASTED CAULIFLOWER WITH SWEET PEPPERS AND CUMIN

Formerly the executive chef at Angelica Kitchen, an organic, vegan restaurant in New York City, Peter Berley, author of *The Modern Vegetarian Kitchen,* is dedicated to organic, vegetarian, seasonal, and sustainable cooking. He has been able to strike a balance between healthy eating and pleasurable eating, as is demonstrated in this Indian-style recipe, which transforms cauliflower from stodgy and boring to vibrant and spicy. Peter suggests serving it with basmati rice or another grain, along with curried chickpeas to create a complete protein.

Another wonderful example of how spices can enhance the taste and digestibility of a vegetable like cauliflower.

Makes 4 servings

3 tablespoons freshly squeezed lemon juice

3 tablespoons extra-virgin olive oil

1½ teaspoons coarse sea salt

1 teaspoon ground cumin

1 teaspoon ground coriander

½ teaspoon cumin seeds

½ teaspoon hot red pepper flakes (Pittas may want to use less)

1 cauliflower (about 2 pounds), cored and separated into florets

1 large red bell pepper, halved, seeded, and sliced into 1-inch-wide strips

1 large yellow bell pepper, halved, seeded, and sliced into 1-inch-wide strips

½ cup fresh cilantro leaves

Preheat the oven to 450 degrees.

In a large bowl, combine the lemon juice, olive oil, salt, ground cumin, coriander, cumin seeds, and red pepper flakes and whisk to combine. Add the cauliflower and bell peppers and toss well.

Spread the vegetables in a baking dish and roast for 45 minutes. Stir every 15 minutes for even browning.

Transfer the vegetables to a serving dish, garnish with the fresh cilantro leaves, and serve.

Per serving: 143 calories; 11 grams fat; 3 grams protein; 11 grams carbohydrate

Nongluten Grains

Grains are always considered a side dish and should be served with a complete protein or with beans to create a complete protein. Vatas can have more grains, and Kaphas should try to restrict themselves to a small portion and have extra vegetables and/or salads.

From Gigia

ROASTED QUINOA VEGETABLE SALAD

Quinoa is an ancient grain grown in the Andes by the Incas. I was thrilled to find it everywhere in my travels to Peru. It contains more essential amino acids than any other grain and is said to be the super-grain of the gods. You'll enjoy its fluffy, nutty quality as an accompaniment to Mexican or Italian dishes.

Quinoa has a bitter coating that can be removed either by soaking it before cooking or by "toasting" it in a dry skillet, which will also give it a nuttier flavor.

Makes 8 servings

1 cup quinoa, rinsed or toasted
2 cups water
1 eggplant, sliced lengthwise
2 zucchini, sliced lengthwise
⅓ cup extra-virgin olive oil
½ pound string beans, washed and
   trimmed

1 onion, cut into ¼-inch rings
4 cloves garlic, peeled and sliced
2 tablespoons balsamic vinegar
¼ cup lemon juice
¼ cup chopped flat-leaf (Italian) parsley
Salt and freshly ground black pepper,
   to taste

Preheat the oven to 350 degrees.

In a dry skillet, lightly toast the quinoa, stirring continuously, until it smells nutty and starts to pop, about 3 to 5 minutes. When done, add the water and cover the pan. Turn the heat to low and steam the grain for 20 to 25 minutes. Remove it from the heat, uncover, and set it aside to cool.

While the quinoa is steaming, lay the eggplant and zucchini slices on a baking sheet, and brush them with half the olive oil. Spread the string beans, onion, and garlic on a second baking sheet, brush them with the remaining oil, and bake all the vegetables in the preheated oven for 30 minutes or until cooked through.

Cut the eggplant and zucchini into thin strips and toss all the vegetables with the quinoa, vinegar, lemon juice, and parsley. Season with salt and pepper to taste and serve warm or at room temperature.

Per serving: 257 calories; 14 grams fat; 6 grams protein; 30 grams carbohydrate

From the Chefs Collaborative: Carrie Balkcom

RISOTTO WITH SAFFRON AND CHEESE

Carrie Balkcom is a member of the national board of overseers for the Chefs Collaborative and runs the Denver chapter. She is one of the spokespeople for the Chefs Collaborative and has dedicated much of her time to educating chefs about the benefits to their restaurants as well as to their clients and the environment of supporting sustainable, organic cuisine. She understands that, given the information, most restaurants are willing to make small changes and do what they can, and she knows that every little bit helps. This dish is great for grounding and nurturing Vatas, especially in the fall and winter. Pittas can enjoy this from time to time, and Kaphas only sparingly.

Makes 6 main course or 8 to 10 side dish servings

¼ cup extra-virgin olive oil
2 tablespoons unsalted butter (use a very good, clear butter, such as Organic Valley)
1 onion, minced
2 cups arborio rice
4 to 5 cups hot chicken or vegetable broth

⅛ teaspoon saffron
6 tablespoons freshly grated Parmesan cheese, plus additional for serving
2 cups coarsely chopped, fresh blanched asparagus*
Salt, to taste

Heat the olive oil and butter in a 6-quart pot over medium heat until the butter is melted. Add the onion and sauté until translucent.

* In place of the asparagus, you can substitute broccoli, fresh mushrooms, carrots, tomatoes, or whatever vegetable is in season and very fresh.

Then add the rice and stir until it absorbs the oil. Add about ½ cup of the hot broth and stir until all the liquid is absorbed. Then add more broth, about ½ cup at a time, stirring after each addition until it is absorbed. When the rice has absorbed 4 cups of the liquid, taste it for tenderness. If it is still hard, add more of the broth and keep cooking and stirring until the rice is tender. Stir in the saffron. (If you are using saffron threads rather than powdered saffron, soak the threads in 2 tablespoons of warm broth before adding them.)

When the saffron is mixed in well, stir in 4 tablespoons of the grated Parmesan. Turn off the heat and let the mixture rest for a few minutes. Then stir in the asparagus until well incorporated. The rice should be creamy and tender. Return it to the heat and heat it through, being careful not to scorch it. Season it with the salt, sprinkle it with the remaining 2 tablespoons of cheese, and pass more at the table.

Per main course serving: 434 calories; 17 grams fat; 16 grams protein; 53 grams carbohydrate

Cook's note: Here in Colorado, we have a wonderful hard goat cheese from Haystack Mountain Goat Dairies that works very well with this dish. We also have a wonderful hard rustic bleu cheese from Bingham Hill Farms that gives this dish a wonderful flavor. If you have local hard cheeses in your area, try them with your fresh local vegetables in this dish.

From Gigia

PESTO POLENTA

Round tubes of ready-made polenta help even the most harried cook serve up this dish with a minimum of effort. Keep a supply of pesto on hand and it will take you just a few minutes. This is so quick and easy that it's one of my favorites. It makes a great hors d'oeuvre or snack to nibble on. Oily, heavy, and grounding, this is another perfect dish for Vatas. Kaphas and others who need to reduce their intake of starchy carbohydrates should indulge only sparingly.

Makes 4 servings

4 to 5 sun-dried tomato halves
1 tablespoon olive oil, for the baking
    sheet

1 package precooked polenta
3 tablespoons pesto (page 252)
¼ cup fresh goat cheese

Preheat the oven to 350 degrees.

Soak the tomato halves in ½ cup of hot water for 10 minutes, then drain and slice them into strips. Oil a baking sheet with the olive oil. Slice 8 pieces of ½-inch-thick polenta and set the slices on the baking sheet. Spread a little of the pesto on each slice of polenta and top the slices with a bit of cheese and a few strips of tomato. Bake 10 minutes, until heated through.

Per serving: 294 calories; 13 grams fat; 12 grams protein; 39 grams carbohydrate

From Gigia

QUINOA WITH CORN TORTILLAS

Making bread without gluten can be daunting, but these simple tortillas are easy. The quinoa adds amino acids as well as a nice nutty flavor.

These small breads can be used for tostadas or eaten as a snack by themselves. You can also bake the cooked tortillas in the oven until crispy and eat them as crackers.

Because these are rather dry and astringent, they will help to decrease Pitta or Kapha. Vatas might want to add some oil and cheese for grounding.

Makes 8 servings

1 cup quinoa flour   Water
1 cup masa harina corn flour   Canola or peanut oil
½ teaspoon salt

Toast the quinoa flour in a dry, heavy skillet over medium-high heat until it turns a few shades darker and starts to give off a nutty aroma. Transfer the quinoa to a mixing bowl, add the masa harina, salt, and about 1 cup of water, just enough to form a thick dough. The dough should come together in a ball without being wet and sticky. Knead it for 2 minutes, until smooth.

Separate the dough into eight 2-inch balls. Roll out the first ball into a thin circle. Heat a skillet over medium-high heat and add ½ teaspoon of oil. When the oil is hot, place the tortilla in the skillet and cook for 2 to 3 minutes until browned. Sprinkle a little oil on top and flip the tortilla. Cook the second side another 2 to 3 minutes, until tender. Repeat the process with the remaining dough.

Per tortilla: 162 calories; 5 grams fat; 4 grams protein; 26 grams carbohydrate

From Gigia

BASMATI RICE

Used in Indian cooking, basmati rice is sweet and cooling; it will help to decrease Pitta or Vata but can increase Kapha if eaten in excess. Using the optional almonds and/or raisins will make the rice even sweeter.

Often, the instructions that come on a package of rice ask for too much water. Basmati is a delicate, long-grained rice that needs only 1½ times as much water as rice (rather than the usual 2 to 1 ratio). By soaking the rice before cooking it, you rinse off the starch, allowing the rice to make a fluffy, chewy pilaf. Brown rice, which is even better for you nutritionally, can be cooked the same way, but you will have to use 2 cups of water and steam it for 45 minutes. You can also buy Lundberg or Fantastic, which are quicker cooking—15 minutes.

Makes 4 servings

1 cup basmati rice
2 teaspoons sesame oil or ghee
½ teaspoon garam masala
1½ cups water

1 teaspoon salt
¼ cup sliced almonds (optional)
¼ cup raisins (optional)

Rinse the rice two or three times, until the water runs clean. Soak the rinsed rice for 10 minutes, then drain it in a wire strainer.

Heat the oil and garam masala in a skillet, and when it is hot, add the rice and sauté it for 3 minutes, until the rice grains are well coated with oil. Add the water and salt and bring the liquid to a boil. Turn the heat down and simmer until most of the water on top of the rice has been absorbed, about 5 minutes. Then cover the pan, turn the heat to low, and steam for 15 minutes. Turn off the heat and let the rice stand, covered, for 5 minutes. Stir in the nuts and/or raisins, if using them, just before serving.

Per serving: 190 calories; 2 grams fat; 4 grams protein; 38 grams carbohydrate

From Gigia

JASMINE RICE

Traditionally used in Thai cooking, jasmine rice has a chewy texture and fragrant aroma that make it the perfect choice when you are serving Asian stir-fries or stews. Make sure you use no more than 1¼ cups of water per cup of rice. An easy way to measure is to put the rice in the saucepan first, then add just enough water to cover the rice by ½ inch. As with all starches, Pittas and Kaphas should not overdo.

Makes 4 servings

1 cup jasmine rice
1¼ cups water

Place the rice in a saucepan and add the water. Cover tightly and bring the water to a boil. As soon as it boils, turn down the heat to the lowest setting. Do not remove the lid or stir the rice. Steam for 15 minutes, then turn off the heat and let the rice sit, covered, for 5 to 10 minutes before serving.

Per serving: 169 calories; less than 1 gram fat; 3 grams protein; 37 grams carbohydrate

Proteins/Main Courses

Remember that it is important to include protein in every meal, to eat no more often than every 3 hours to allow time for digestion, and no less often than every 3½ hours to avoid the blood sugar swings that will lead to those cravings for sweets and starchy carbohydrates.

From Gigia

TOFU-AND-BROCCOLI STIR-FRY

Use this basic recipe to create any stir-fry you wish. Traditionally, the meat or protein is quickly stir-fried first, then removed from the pan. Once that is done, add the flavorings, such as chilies, garlic, or ginger. After a few quick stirs, begin adding the vegetables, starting with those that take longest to cook. Laying out the ingredients close to hand before you start helps to keep the stir-fry hopping.

Pittas should probably use less of the heating chili paste in the sauce than either Vatas or Kaphas. And remember to pay attention to your body. Both tofu and broccoli can be hard on Vata digestion.

For the Stir-Fry

1 package firm tofu
1 bunch green onions
4 tablespoons vegetable oil
1 tablespoon minced ginger
4 cloves garlic, sliced

2 heads broccoli, cut into long
    flowerets
1 red bell pepper, seeded and cut into
    strips

For the Sauce

1 tablespoon cornstarch
⅓ cup Chinese cooking wine
3 tablespoons Chinese soy sauce or
    wheat-free tamari
⅓ cup vegetable stock or 1 teaspoon
    miso mixed with ⅓ cup water

2 teaspoons chili paste
2 tablespoons black bean sauce
    (optional)
1 tablespoon sugar
½ teaspoon salt
1½ tablespoons toasted sesame oil

Cut the tofu into ½-inch cubes and place it between paper towels. Set a weight (like a cutting board) on top and let the tofu sit while you prepare the vegetables and combine the ingredients for the sauce in a bowl and set aside.

Cut the ends off the green onions, cut them into 2-inch lengths, and shred each piece lengthwise so that you have long, thin strands of onion.

When all the ingredients are prepared, heat a wok or skillet and add 4 tablespoons of the vegetable oil. When the oil is hot, add the tofu, a few pieces at a time, and stir-fry until golden brown and slightly puffed. Remove the tofu with a slotted spoon as it is done and transfer it to paper towels to drain. When all the tofu is done, drain some of the oil from the pan and add the ginger and garlic. Stir a few times and add the broccoli. Cover the wok or skillet for 1 minute and remove the lid. The broccoli should be bright green. Add the red pepper and cook 1 to 2 minutes. Return the tofu to the pan and stir the ingredients together. Then add the sauce. When the sauce is thickened, add the green onion and stir for 1 minute. Serve at once over rice.

Per serving: 250 calories; 17 grams fat; 10 grams protein; 19 grams carbohydrate

From Jennifer

QUICK AND EASY MARINATED TOFU

You can also use this marinade to make quick and easy chicken, shrimp, or fish. Remember that too much tofu can increase Kapha and be difficult for Vatas to digest. Nevertheless, this is a great recipe if you don't overdo.

Makes 2 servings

1 tablespoon chopped fresh ginger   2 tablespoons honey
1 teaspoon toasted sesame oil   ½ package firm tofu
2 tablespoons wheat-free tamari

Preheat the oven to 350 degrees.

Combine the ginger, sesame oil, tamari, and honey. Slice the tofu into ½-inch-thick rectangles—you should have about 3 or 4 pieces. Place it in a baking dish and pour the marinade over it. Bake in the preheated oven for 20 to 30 minutes, or until all the liquid is gone. Serve the tofu over a small quantity of rice, with lots of vegetables to go with it.

Per serving: 211 calories; 9 grams fat; 14 grams protein; 23 grams carbohydrate

From the Chefs Collaborative: Michael Romano

STUFFED CHICKEN BREASTS WITH HERBED GOAT CHEESE

Michael Romano, his partner, Danny Meyer, and their restaurant, the Union Square Café, are without doubt one of the most beloved and admired culinary trios in the United States. In 1985, when Meyer was searching for the perfect location for his restaurant, the nearby Union Square green market's promise of "fantastic produce" was a major selling point. Since then, says Romano, "our main focus is working with the farmer's market at Union Square. We feel it is an important way [to] support local agriculture. We support our farmers [and] we support the principle of sustainability because we are using what is in season, locally grown."

Executive chef Michael Romano has been kind enough to allow us to reprint this recipe from *The Union Square Café Cookbook*. To quote from the introduction to this recipe in the book, "Our chickens are always free range and certified organic, and our goat cheese is from a local producer. It is important to maintain a connection with people of integrity who grow clean quality food."

This is good for all three constitutional types, although some Kaphas might find it a bit too heavy.

Makes 4 servings

4 ounces fresh, soft goat cheese (½ cup)
1 tablespoon each, minced tarragon, basil, parsley, and chives
3 tablespoons extra-virgin olive oil
¼ teaspoon kosher salt

Freshly ground black pepper
4 boneless chicken breasts, with a 3-inch-long pocket cut into the thickest part—have your butcher do this for you

In a bowl, thoroughly combine the goat cheese, herbs, 1 tablespoon olive oil, and half the salt and pepper. Using your fingers, or a small spoon, stuff a quarter of the filling into each breast. Close each pocket with a toothpick. Season the breasts with the remaining salt and pepper, cover, and refrigerate for 1 hour or up to a day ahead.

Heat the remaining olive oil over medium-high heat in a 10-inch skillet. Place the stuffed chicken breasts skin side down in the pan. Sauté 5 to 6 minutes, until golden brown. Using a spatula, turn over and cook an additional 3 to 5 minutes, or until the chicken is somewhat firm to the touch. Transfer the breasts to a warm platter, remove the toothpicks, and serve.

Per serving: 323 calories; 22 grams fat; 29 grams protein; 1 gram carbohydrate

From Gigia

TEMPEH STICKS

Because tempeh is a cake of whole, fermented soybeans, it has more inherent texture than tofu. It can be crumbled and used as a substitute for ground beef in tacos or sloppy joes. Steaming or blanching the tempeh in broth before cooking will help to make it more digestible. Enjoy tempeh sticks as an appetizer served with peanut sauce, or serve them with rice and steamed vegetables as a main course.

These are great as an after-school treat for kids or an after-work snack for grown-ups. Just pay attention to how you're digesting the soy and don't overdo it. This recipe is perfect for Vatas and Pittas. The coconut milk, sugar, and lime juice will balance the heating quality of the peanuts. Kaphas should eat this in smaller amounts.

Makes 4 servings as a main course or 8 as an appetizer

8 ounces tempeh
1 teaspoon salt
3 cloves garlic

1½ teaspoons ground coriander
2 tablespoons canola oil
Peanut sauce (optional), recipe follows

Cut the tempeh into ⅜-inch-wide strips. In a bowl large enough to hold the tempeh, combine the salt, garlic, and coriander. Heat the canola oil in a wok or skillet over medium heat. While the oil is heating, add the tempeh to the bowl with the seasoning and stir to coat well. Remove the sticks a few at a time, and add them to the hot oil. Stir-fry for 3 to 5 minutes or until the tempeh is golden to reddish brown and crisp. Remove the sticks with a slotted spoon and transfer to drain on paper towels. Continue to add and stir-fry until all the tempeh is done.

Per appetizer serving: 88 calories; 6 grams fat; 5 grams protein; 5 grams carbohydrate

From Gigia

PEANUT SAUCE

Serve this with the tempeh sticks (above) for a tangy Indonesian snack. It's also delicious over brown rice and steamed vegetables.

Makes 16 servings

3 whole serrano peppers
4 cloves garlic
¼ cup dry-roasted, unsalted peanuts
4 teaspoons soy sauce or fish sauce
4 teaspoons lime juice
4 teaspoons brown sugar or palm
   sugar

4 teaspoons tamarind pulp
2 tablespoons coconut milk
2 tablespoons plus 2 teaspoons water
Chopped fresh cilantro, for garnish

In a blender, combine all the ingredients except the cilantro and add 2 tablespoons plus 2 teaspoons of water. Blend until smooth.

Transfer the sauce to a small bowl and garnish it with the cilantro.

Per serving: 23 calories; 1 gram fat; 1 gram protein; 3 grams carbohydrate

From the Chefs Collaborative: Nora Pouillon

PORTOBELLO MUSHROOM CURRY WITH LEMON BASMATI RICE

Nora Pouillon is chef/owner of Nora and Asia Nora in Washington, D.C. When Nora became the first certified organic restaurant in the country, it was the culmination of years spent seeking out and working with local farmers and buying seasonal foods. "Today," Nora says, "with greater awareness toward the quality of our food, and the growth of organic farming, it is possible to run a certified organic restaurant offering a sophisticated cuisine using the purest ingredients available." She hopes that other chefs will be encouraged to go organic as well. Nora is truly an inspiration and an amazing woman.

A good recipe for all three types, although Pittas may need to reduce the quantity of chilies. Kaphas would do well to go easy on the rice.

Makes 4 servings

For the Mushroom Curry

1 (4-inch) piece of ginger, peeled and sliced across the grain

2 whole jalapeño or serrano chilies, steamed

1 cup vegetable stock or water

4 tablespoons canola oil

1½ pounds onions, minced (about 2 large onions)

1 tablespoon minced garlic

3 tablespoons good-quality curry powder, available at specialty stores

1 cup low-fat yogurt

Sea salt and freshly ground black pepper

2 pounds portobello mushrooms, cleaned and cut into 1½-inch pieces

2 teaspoons garam masala, available at specialty stores

1 tablespoon lemon juice (optional)

½ cup chopped cilantro

Put the ginger, chilies, and vegetable stock or water in a blender and puree until smooth.

Heat 2 tablespoons of the canola oil in a sauté pan or casserole large enough to hold all the ingredients. Sauté the onions over low heat, stirring frequently for 15 to 20 minutes, or until they are soft and golden. Add the garlic and the curry powder and stir and sauté for about 2 more minutes. Add the ginger-chili mixture and yogurt and season to taste with salt and pepper. This is the base sauce for your curry.

Heat the remaining oil in a sauté pan and brown the mushrooms, stirring for 2 to 3 minutes. Transfer them into the curry base. Bring to a boil, add the garam masala and simmer until the mushrooms are tender.

Just before serving the curry, add the optional lemon juice and the cilantro.

Per serving: 221 calories; 4 grams fat; 13 grams protein; 39 grams carbohydrate

For the Basmati Rice

3 cups water
2 cups basmati rice, available at health food or specialty stores, or use other long-grain rice

½ teaspoon sea salt
Grated peel of 1 lemon

Bring the water to a boil in a medium saucepan. Add the rice, salt, and lemon peel. Bring back to a boil, stirring to combine, lower the heat, and cover. Simmer over a very low flame for about 14 minutes or until the rice is tender.

Uncover the rice and stir with a fork to plump the rice and separate the grains.

Per serving: 341 calories; less than 1 gram fat; 7 grams protein; 76 grams carbohydrate

From Jennifer

RICE CRUST PIZZA

This is great for kids, especially if they have food allergies or sensitivities to wheat, gluten, or dairy. And it's also a good thing for adults to serve on Super Bowl Sunday, or any other football game–watching afternoon or evening.

Great for Vatas and Pittas. Still a bit heavy—although lighter than regular pizza—for Kaphas.

Makes 2 adult servings

4 tablespoons Garden Valley tomato sauce

2 tablespoons pesto (page 252)

1 rice pizza crust*

¼ cup chopped frozen spinach or sautéed vegetables (see sautéed kale, page 213)

2 Roma tomatoes or 6 sun-dried tomato halves

¼ cup goat's milk mozzarella cheese

2 tablespoons crumbled feta cheese

Preheat the oven to 400 degrees.

Spread the tomato sauce and pesto over the pizza crust. Add the spinach and tomatoes. Sprinkle the cheese over all. Bake in the preheated oven until the top of the pizza is brown and bubbly.

Per serving: 389 calories; 13 grams fat; 13 grams protein; 55 grams carbohydrate

* Nature's Hilights makes this. You can buy it at health food stores.

SPICY GRILLED SHRIMP STEW (Caldo de Camarón Asado)

The warm and friendly atmosphere of Rick Bayless's two Chicago restaurants, Topolobampo and the Frontera Grill, perfectly reflects his kind and generous spirit. They serve the authentic Mexican cuisine that has won him not only culinary prizes, but an international reputation as well. In addition to being a world-class chef, he has served as president of the Chefs Collaborative and is a prolific cookbook writer as well. He is dedicated to educating his customers and other chefs and restaurateurs about the rewards of championing sustainable, seasonal, local, organic products in support of a more environmentally friendly food delivery system.

The recipe here is reprinted from Rick's most recent book, *Mexico: One Plate at a Time.* He is also the host of a PBS cooking series of the same name.

This recipe is good for all three constitutional types. Vatas can have more of the potatoes, and Pittas might get a bit overheated from the tomatoes.

Makes 6 generous servings

1 small white onion, sliced ¼ inch thick

3 garlic cloves, peeled and roughly chopped

1½ pounds (9 to 12 plum or 3 medium-large round) ripe tomatoes, roughly chopped

or

1 (28-ounce) can good-quality whole tomatoes in juice, drained

2 tablespoons olive oil, preferably extra-virgin, plus additional for brushing or spraying the shrimp and vegetables

6 cups good chicken broth, store-bought or homemade

1 to 2 large sprigs fresh epazote (or a small handful fresh cilantro or parsley, if no epazote is at hand, plus a few sprigs for garnish)

2 pounds (about 48) medium shrimp

12 bamboo skewers, about 7 inches long, soaked in water at least 20 minutes

Salt

About 2 tablespoons pure ground chili (preferably ancho or guajillo chili, though New Mexico chili will do nicely)

3 medium (about 1½ pounds) sweet potatoes (I especially like the purple-skin Mexican sweet potatoes called camotes morados), peeled and sliced ½ inch thick

or

3 medium chayotes (about 2 pounds), halved, pit removed, and sliced ½ inch thick

or

3 large (about 1½ pounds) Yukon gold potatoes, sliced ½ inch thick

In a blender or food processor, combine the onion and garlic with the tomatoes. Process to a smooth puree. In a medium-size (4-to-5-quart) pot (preferably a Dutch oven or Mexican *cazuela*), heat the oil over medium-high. When hot enough to make a drop of the puree sizzle sharply, add it all at once and stir continually until darker in color and cooked down to the consistency of tomato paste, 10 to 12 minutes. Stir in the broth and epazote (or one of its stand-ins). Partially cover and simmer over medium-low heat for about 30 minutes.

While the broth is simmering, peel the shrimp, leaving their final joint and tail intact. Devein each shrimp by making a shallow incision down the back and scraping out what is usually a dark, veinlike intestinal tract. Impale the shrimp on the skewers (about 4 on each), being careful not to bunch them too tightly. Lay them out flat on a tray and sprinkle them on both sides with salt and ground chili.

To finish the dish, heat a gas grill to medium or light a charcoal fire and let it burn until the coals are covered with gray ash and medium hot. Taste the broth and season it with salt, usually about ¾ teaspoon; keep warm, covered, over low heat. Generously brush or spray the sliced sweet potato, chayote, or potato with olive oil, sprinkle both sides of each piece with salt, and grill, turning occasionally, until soft through, 10 to 15 minutes. Divide among 6 large soup bowls.

Lightly brush or spray the shrimp with olive oil and lay them on the grill. Cook until just done through, 2 to 3 minutes per side.

Ladle the steaming broth over the vegetables in each soup bowl. Lay 2 skewers of shrimp in each bowl (they'll rise dramatically from the broth, toward the edge of the bowls). Garnish with an herb sprig and you're ready to present this dramatic, lusty soup to your guests.

Per serving: 366 calories; 11 grams fat; 44 grams protein; 23 grams carbohydrate

From Gigia

TANDOORI SALMON

Cold-water fish such as salmon provide a good source of protein and essential fatty acids. Look for wild salmon from Alaska. Farm-raised salmon may have been subject to genetic engineering and may contain pollutants and/or dyes, so check with your supplier about the source of your fish.

This is a good recipe for all three constitutional types. Vatas might want a grounding side dish to go with it.

Makes 4 servings

Juice of 1 lemon
1½ pounds salmon fillets
Salt, to taste
1 cup plain yogurt
1 (1-inch) piece fresh ginger, peeled
   and chopped
2 cloves garlic, chopped
1 jalapeño pepper, chopped
1 teaspoon whole black peppercorns
1 teaspoon garam masala
½ teaspoon turmeric
Fresh cilantro or mint, for garnish
4 lemon wedges, for garnish

Pour the lemon juice over the salmon and rub it with salt.

Combine the yogurt, ginger, garlic, jalapeño, black peppercorns, garam masala, and turmeric in a blender and blend until smooth. Spoon this mixture over the salmon and refrigerate it for at least 4, or up to 8, hours.

Preheat the oven to 500 degrees and bake the salmon for 10 minutes, until it flakes easily with a fork. Garnish it with sprigs of cilantro or mint and serve it with the lemon wedges.

Per serving: 259 calories; 7 grams fat; 38 grams protein; 11 grams carbohydrate

From the Chefs Collaborative: Tim Keating

PAN-SEARED TRUE AMERICAN RED SNAPPER, PROVENÇALE VEGETABLES, ARTICHOKE-AND-FENNEL NAGE

Executive chef at the Four Seasons Hotel in Houston, Texas, Tim Keating has been a member of the national executive committee of the Chefs Collaborative since 1996. He says that "dealing with local farmers gives us all a great sense of community, and watching many of them here in Houston grow and prosper gives us great satisfaction."

Makes 4 servings

For the Nage

4 large artichokes
Fresh lemon juice
Pinch of kosher salt
1 ounce olive and canola oil blend
1 small onion, sliced
2 leeks, white and some green part, sliced

1 medium fennel bulb, chopped
2 Roma tomatoes, chopped
2 elephant garlic cloves, sliced
½ teaspoon fennel seeds, toasted and coarsely chopped
1 cup dry white wine
5 cups water

For the Fish and Garnish

4 (5-ounce) red snapper fillets, skin on
Fresh ground pepper, to taste
Olive oil/canola oil cooking spray
4 Roma tomatoes, peeled and split in quarters
½ teaspoon chopped garlic
½ teaspoon chopped lemon thyme
1 roasted red pepper, deseeded and julienned
4 tiny artichokes, turned, blanched, and cut in half

4 small red creamer potatoes, roasted and cut in half
2 ounces haricots verts, blanched and shocked
8 tiny squash, blanched and shocked
8 tiny pearl onions, peeled and blanched
12 bias-cut zucchini slices, blanched
16 calamata, gaeta, or Provence olives, pitted
Fresh herbs (basil, oregano, etc.), for garnish

To make the nage: Peel the artichokes down to the choke, discarding the leaves and trimming to reach the heart, the rounded base of the artichoke. Scrape away the fuzzy choke and immerse the artichokes in water acidulated with a bit of lemon juice and salt to prevent discoloration. In a medium saucepan, heat the oil and add the onion, leeks, fennel, tomatoes, garlic, and fennel seeds. Sauté for 8 to 10 minutes, until all are translucent. Add the white wine and cook for 5 to 6 minutes. Add the water, bring to a slow rolling boil, and cook for 30 minutes. Strain through a fine mesh strainer, return the liquid to the heat, and reduce by half. Set aside and reserve.

To make the snapper: Season the fish with fresh ground pepper and sauté it, skin side down, in a preheated medium-size skillet sprayed with a scant olive/canola oil mist. Be sure the skin is crisp before turning to cook the other side for just 20 seconds. Transfer the fish to a 350-degree oven and bake for 6 to 8 minutes, until firm to the touch. Place the tomatoes in a small skillet, season them with the garlic and thyme, and roast in a 350-degree oven for 10 minutes. Set aside and reserve. In a separate skillet coated with canola/olive oil mist, reheat all the blanched vegetables until just heated, moving the pan continuously. Add a bit of the nage to the pan if it gets too dry. Arrange the blanched vegetables, potatoes, tomatoes, red pepper, and olives in the base of a large bowl and top with the roasted snapper. Moisten each serving with 2 ounces of the nage and garnish the dish with the herbs.

Per serving: 573 calories; 13 grams fat; 44 grams protein; 71 grams carbohydrate

From the Chefs Collaborative: Ron Pickarski

MOO GOO GAI PAN

Ron Pickarski is dedicated to seeing vegetarianism reach the esteemed state of haute cuisine by translating classical meat-based cuisine into vegetarian cuisine, and to helping Americans introduce more whole foods and vegetarian dishes into their diet. That is the premise of his book, the *As You Like It Cookbook* (Square One Publishers), which offers traditional dishes and follows them with vegetarian alternatives. The following recipe is taken from that book.

Great for Pittas and Kaphas, this is light and easy to digest.

Makes 4 servings

1 tablespoon plain (not roasted) sesame oil
1 pound thinly sliced chicken breast
2 cups thinly sliced onions
2 cups quartered mushrooms
2 cups thinly sliced red and/or green bell peppers

2 cups thinly sliced Napa cabbage
1 cup thinly sliced bok choy
1 cup mung bean sprouts
1 cup sliced water chestnuts
2 cups moo goo gai pan sauce (recipe follows)

Heat the sesame oil in a wok or a large, deep skillet over medium-high heat. Add the chicken and stir-fry about 3 minutes, or until lightly browned.

Add the vegetables and continue to stir-fry for 3 to 5 minutes, or until the vegetables are tender-crisp. Add the sauce and simmer. Serve immediately over rice.

Per serving (without rice, sauce included): 434 calories; 26 grams fat; 23 grams protein; 25 grams carbohydrate

Vegan choice: Replace the chicken with ½-inch cubes of extra-firm tofu that have been sprinkled with tamari or other soy sauce. You can also replace the chicken with seitan or a vegetarian chicken alternative.

Moo Goo Gai Pan Sauce

¼ cup sesame oil

4½ teaspoons minced fresh ginger

4½ teaspoons minced fresh garlic

2 cups water

¼ cup sherry wine

1½ teaspoons sea salt

⅛ teaspoon white pepper

3 tablespoons arrowroot

Heat the sesame oil in a 1-quart saucepan over medium heat. Add the ginger and garlic, and sauté for about 3 minutes, or until they are soft but not browned. Add the water, wine, salt, and pepper, and stir well. Bring to a simmer, then turn off the heat. Stir in the arrowroot, turn the heat to medium, and continue to stir for 3 to 5 minutes, or until the sauce has thickened. Use immediately or transfer to a covered container and store in the refrigerator, where it will keep for about 1 week.

From Indira

MUNG DAHL

Mung dahl, or kichadi, is a staple dish in Ayurvedic cooking and extremely easy to digest. For cleansing purposes, the soupier it is, the better. And if you serve this over or with basmati rice, it becomes an excellent source of complete protein for vegetarians. Pittas might want to use less ginger and garlic and more cilantro than are called for in this recipe. *Fresh* ginger is actually good for Pittas. It's also great for Vatas and easy to digest.

Makes 4 servings

½ cup split yellow mung beans
6 to 7 cups water
2 tablespoons ghee* or oil
Pinch of asafoetida (hing)
½ teaspoon cumin seeds
2 teaspoons finely chopped fresh ginger

2 teaspoons finely chopped garlic
¼ teaspoon turmeric
Salt, to taste
2 tablespoons fresh lemon juice
2 to 3 tablespoons chopped cilantro
2 tablespoons finely chopped tomato or red bell pepper

* Ghee, or clarified butter from which the milk solids have been removed, is another staple of Ayurvedic cooking and preferred to butter by many chefs as well. In Ayurvedic cooking it is used as a carrier to help herbs and spices enter the tissues, and it is also used to remove blockages. Where regular butter "clogs," ghee does not. It will help to increase *ojas* and is recommended for Vatas and Pittas; Kaphas should use it in smaller amounts.

To make ghee: Place ½ pound of organic sweet butter at room temperature in a medium saucepan. Put it on the smallest burner of your stove and cook on low heat for 25 minutes. *Do not stir.* Keep the pot partially covered to avoid splattering. In about 20 minutes you will notice a light brown residue emerging from the bottom of the pot among the froth and foam. Continue to cook another 5 minutes, until the butter is a clear golden color and has a nutty aroma. Remove from the heat and cool to lukewarm. Then strain to remove the white milk solids and continue to cool completely. Store in a cool, dry place. Properly clarified, ghee will last a few months without refrigeration. Use it with a pinch of sea salt to sauté or flavor vegetables.

Wash the beans and soak them for several hours. Bring the water to a boil in a large pot, and boil the beans for 15 minutes. Reduce the heat and simmer for 1 hour, then mash the beans until smooth (a rice masher does a good job of this).

In a small skillet, heat the ghee over medium heat and add the asafetida and cumin seeds. Let them sizzle for a few seconds, then stir in the ginger and garlic. Cook for 2 or 3 minutes, then pour over the beans. Add all the remaining ingredients and heat through.

Per serving: 156 calories; 7 grams fat; 7 grams protein; 18 grams carbohydrate

From the Chefs Collaborative: Stan Frankenthaler

STIR-FRY SHRIMP AND LITTLENECK CLAMS IN A SWEET-AND-SOUR ORGANIC TOMATO BROTH

Stan Frankenthaler, who kindly contributed this recipe, is the chef/ owner of Salamander Restaurant in Cambridge, Massachusetts, where he serves a unique, Asian-inspired fusion cuisine, which is reflected in the Southeast Asian flavors of this broth.

A member of the board of overseers of the Chefs Collaborative, he worked in partnership with the Environmental Protection Agency to create a guide called *Seafood Solutions,* to educate chefs and restaurateurs about ecologically responsible fish procurement.

Chef Frankenthaler uses Muir Glen canned tomatoes for their flavor, quality, and consistency. Using them makes it possible for you to create this dish in any season of the year.

This wonderful recipe is light and easy to digest. It's great for Kaphas but may be a bit heating for Pittas.

Serves 6 as an appetizer or luncheon dish

For the Broth

1 tablespoon dark sesame oil
1 large onion, diced
1 stalk lemongrass, trimmed and
    minced
1 tablespoon minced fresh ginger
1 tablespoon minced garlic
2 cups fish fumet or vegetable
    broth
⅓ cup rice vinegar

¼ cup mirin
2 tablespoons tamari
1 cup diced fresh organic
    pineapple
1 tablespoon tamarind pulp
1 (28-ounce) can Muir Glen diced
    tomatoes
1 teaspoon ground coriander
Salt and pepper, to taste

For the Seafood

12 littleneck clams
1 tablespoon minced fresh ginger
1 tablespoon minced fresh garlic

8 ounces fresh, local shrimp (or best
    quality you can get)
1 tablespoon light sesame oil

For the Garnishes

6 fresh sprigs cilantro
6 fresh sprigs mint

6 lime wedges

To make the broth: Heat the dark sesame oil and sauté the onion, lemongrass, ginger, and garlic 4 to 5 minutes, until lightly caramelized. Then add all the liquids, the pineapple, tamarind, and tomatoes. Bring to a boil, season with the coriander and salt and pepper, and simmer 15 to 20 minutes. The broth can be made 1 to 2 days ahead, refrigerated, and reheated before serving.

To make the seafood: Wash the clams thoroughly under cold running water and steam them open in the broth. Quickly, in a very hot pan, sauté the ginger, garlic, and shrimp in the light sesame oil.

Ladle the broth into warm soup plates, place two clams in each bowl, and ladle the sautéed shrimp over them. Garnish with the cilantro and mint sprigs and the lime wedges.

Per serving: 221 calories; 8 grams fat; 14 grams protein; 21 grams carbohydrate

From Gigia

PAN-FRIED CHICKEN BREASTS

Skinless and boneless chicken breasts can be dry and unappealing, but if you pan-fry them in a little olive oil, and if you're careful not to overcook them, they will be moist and juicy. If you like, you can add a splash of wine or brandy to the pan and let the liquid cook off for a really juicy fillet. (See "Variations" below.) Make extra while you're at it, because these are also great for sandwiches and in a noodle bowl.

Light and good for all three constitutional types. Kaphas should have this with lots of vegetables, too.

Makes 4 servings

4 skinless and boneless chicken breasts (preferably free range and organic)

2 tablespoons olive oil
Salt and freshly ground pepper, to taste
½ lemon

Rinse the chicken under cold running water and pat it dry. Remove the small fillet on the back of each breast by peeling it off with your fingers. Cut off the tough white tendon in the middle of the small fillet. Trim any remaining skin or fat from the breasts and, if you have a meat mallet, pound them lightly (being careful not to tear the meat) until they flatten out. Rub them with 1 tablespoon of the olive oil.

Heat a dry heavy skillet for 5 minutes on medium-high heat. Add the remaining olive oil to the pan and then the breasts and fillets. Let the breasts cook without moving them for at least 5 minutes, to brown on the bottom. Then sprinkle them with salt and pepper, turn them over, and cook another 3 to 5 minutes. The fillets will be done a few minutes before the breasts. You can tell the chicken is done when it is firm but still gives to the touch. Don't overcook it or it will dry out. When done, remove the breasts to a platter and squeeze the juice of the ½ lemon over them.

Per serving: 185 calories; 8 grams fat; 26 grams protein; 1 gram carbohydrate

Variations: You can sprinkle the breasts with dried herbs such as rosemary, sage, or thyme, or rub them with chili or curry powder before cooking. After cooking, with the chicken still in the pan, you can pour in ¼ cup of wine and let it boil off, infusing the chicken with the wine.

From the Chefs Collaborative: Alice Waters

RARE YELLOWFIN TUNA WITH CORIANDER AND FENNEL SEED

Alice Waters is the visionary chef and owner of Chez Panisse in Berkeley, California. She is the author of four cookbooks, including *Chez Panisse Vegetables* and *Fanny at Chez Panisse*. In 1994 she founded the Edible Schoolyard in Berkeley's Martin Luther King, Jr., Middle School, a model curriculum that integrates organic gardening into academic classes and into the life of the school; it will soon incorporate a school lunch program in which students will prepare, serve, and share food they grow themselves, augmented by organic dairy products, grains, fruits, vegetables, meat, and fish—all locally and sustainably produced.

This recipe is from the *Chez Panisse Café Cookbook*.

Makes 6 to 8 servings

2 pounds center-cut tuna	Cracked black pepper
3 to 4 tablespoons olive oil	2 tablespoons coriander seeds
Salt	1 tablespoon fennel seeds

For the Vinaigrette and Garnish

3 small shallots, diced fine	1 medium fennel bulb, trimmed
Juice of ½ lemon	1 small bunch radishes, trimmed
3 tablespoons champagne vinegar	1 small bunch cilantro, tough stems
Salt	removed
½ cup extra-virgin olive oil	

Ask your fishmonger for 2 pieces of tuna weighing 1 pound each, the pieces about 3 inches in diameter and 8 inches long. Rub the tuna fillets with olive oil and season generously with salt and cracked pepper. In a mortar, crush the coriander and fennel seeds coarsely, until their fragrance is released. Sprinkle the crushed seeds evenly over the tuna, pressing them into the flesh. This can be done several hours before cooking. Hold in the refrigerator.

Heat a large cast-iron skillet over medium-high heat until almost smoking. Carefully place the seasoned tuna in the skillet and sear for

30 seconds on each side. Remove the tuna to a platter and cool for an hour or so at room temperature.

Make the vinaigrette by macerating the shallots in the lemon juice and champagne vinegar with a good pinch of salt for 10 minutes. Whisk in the olive oil, taste, and adjust the seasoning.

Use a very sharp knife to slice the tuna into even ⅛-inch slices. Place 2 slices side by side on each serving plate. Using a Japanese mandolin, shave the fennel bulb into thin ribbons and strew them over the fish. Shave some radish slices and strew them over the fish in the same way. The result should be a playful mosaic effect. Splash the vinaigrette over the tuna, fennel, and radishes. Add a light sprinkling of salt. Roughly chop the cilantro, scatter it over each plate, and serve.

Per serving (for 6 servings, using all the vinaigrette): 460 calories; 32 grams fat; 36 grams protein; 5 grams carbohydrate

From the Chefs Collaborative: Greg Higgins

BROILED PAVE OF HALIBUT WITH CITRUS COUS-COUS, RED ONION MARMALADE, AND CILANTRO-ALMOND SAUCE

Greg Higgins, of the nationally renowned Higgins Restaurant in Portland, Oregon, has made it his business to establish connections with the local farming community that allow him to give his clientele the freshest of locally grown ingredients, artfully prepared and beautifully presented.

A member of the board of overseers of the Chefs Collaborative, he worked with Stan Frankenthaler as a contributor to *Seafood Solutions*.

Pittas might want to cool down the sauce by using a somewhat smaller quantity of jalapeños.

Makes 1 serving

For the Red Onion Marmalade

½ cup port wine
¼ cup red wine vinegar
¼ cup sugar

Zest and juice of 1 orange
2 cups julienned red onion
Salt and pepper, to taste

Bring the wine, vinegar, sugar, and orange juice to a boil in a non-reactive saucepan and boil for 7 to 10 minutes, until reduced by ⅓ to a light syrup. Add the orange zest and onion and cook until al dente, about 3 to 5 minutes. Adjust the seasonings with salt and pepper to taste.

For the Cilantro-Almond Sauce

1 bunch cilantro, washed and chopped	½ cup toasted sliced almonds
	1 teaspoon cumin
2 jalapeño peppers, seeded and chopped	2 tablespoons honey
	¼ cup fresh lime juice
1 tablespoon minced garlic	Salt and pepper, to taste

Puree all the ingredients except the salt and pepper in a blender, adding water if needed to thin the mixture slightly to a pourable consistency. Season to taste with salt and pepper. The sauce should have a nutty, spicy, aromatic character.

For the Citrus Cous-Cous

Juice and zest of 1 orange	½ teaspoon ground turmeric or curry powder
Juice and zest of 1 lemon	
2 tablespoons minced garlic	1¾ cups water
1 tablespoon chili paste (Sambal Oelek)	Salt and pepper, to taste
	2 cups uncooked cous-cous*

Chop the citrus zests and combine them with the garlic, chili paste, spices, citrus juices, and water. Bring the mixture to a boil and season to taste with salt and pepper. Put the cous-cous in a shallow pan and pour the seasoning mixture over it. Cover the pan with plastic wrap and let it sit for 5 to 10 minutes. Fluff the cous-cous with a fork, and keep it warm until ready to serve.

* To make this a gluten-free dish, you can substitute quinoa for the cous-cous.

For the Broiled Pave of Halibut

1 (4-to-6-ounce) pave (square cut)
    fillet of halibut, or any other flaky
    white-fleshed fish
1 tablespoon Madras curry powder

1 tablespoon kosher salt
Olive oil in a mister or vegetable oil
    cooking spray
4 ounces fresh salad greens (mesclun)

Season the halibut with the curry powder and salt. Mist it lightly with the oil. Char-broil or pan-sear the fish in a nonstick pan 2 to 3 minutes on each side, or until just firm. Serve on the cous-cous and greens, surrounded by the cilantro-almond sauce and topped with the marmalade.

Per serving: 584 calories; 11 grams fat; 38 grams protein; 81 grams carbohydrate

Dressings, Chutneys, and Relishes

Use these to be sure you're getting all six tastes in every meal, to satisfy your taste buds, and to keep your body and mind in balance. They provide lots of flavor with very few calories. If you think you don't have time to make your own, consider trying one or more of the delicious premade chutneys and other ethnic flavorings on page 286.

From Gigia

LOW-FAT RANCH DRESSING

Silken tofu is an excellent nondairy option for creamy dressing and desserts. If you have trouble digesting vinegars, this dressing may be the answer for you, as it was for many of my clients.

Great for Vatas who don't have a problem digesting soy, and also good for Pittas. Kaphas should use this sparingly.

Makes 24 servings

2 tablespoons miso
2 cups water
10 ounces light silken tofu
1 teaspoon salt
2 tablespoons fresh lemon juice

2 tablespoons chopped fresh chives
1 tablespoon chopped fresh parsley
½ teaspoon freshly ground black
    pepper

Combine the miso, water, tofu, salt, and lemon juice in a blender and blend until smooth. Add the herbs and pepper and stir to combine.

Per serving: 8 calories; less than 1 gram of fat; 1 gram protein; 1 gram carbohydrate

Variations: You can also add poppy seeds, crushed toasted sesame seeds, or garlic to the dressing, according to your taste.

From Gigia

MISO DRESSING

This tangy dressing adds zip and flavor to salads, sandwiches, and steamed vegetables. Because it's made with very little oil, it's very low in fat.

Light and good for all three types.

Makes 12 servings

1 tablespoon white or yellow miso	1 teaspoon sesame oil
2 tablespoons fresh lemon juice	2 teaspoons honey or palm sugar
1 tablespoon toasted sesame seeds	

Combine all the ingredients in a bowl and whisk together with a fork.

Per serving: 15 calories; 1 gram fat; 1 gram protein; 2 grams carbohydrate

Variations: Use orange or lime juice instead of the lemon juice. Add ginger, garlic, cilantro, or mint to your taste.

From Gigia

PESTO

Many people find it difficult to digest "restaurant" pestos because they tend to be rather heavy. This is pesto stripped to the basics: olive oil, basil, and garlic. In Ayurveda, basil is a very powerful, healing plant, and when used in combination with these other ingredients, it is full of *prana* and is healing and grounding.

Add cheese, if you wish, to your noodles, but not to the pesto. The hot noodles will make the pesto clump together if there is cheese in it. You can also add a tablespoon of miso instead of the salt, which will give the pesto a creamy texture. Freeze the pesto in ice cube trays to have it on hand for small servings whenever you wish.

Especially good for Vatas and Kaphas. Pittas can cut down on the garlic if they find it too stimulating.

2 cups fresh basil leaves   ¼ cup olive oil
3 cloves garlic   Lemon juice, to taste (optional)
½ teaspoon sea salt

Combine the basil, garlic, and salt in a blender, and pulse to chop the basil leaves. Then add the olive oil slowly, blending after each addition, until you have a thick, green paste. If you like, you can add lemon juice to brighten the flavor and cut down on the amount of oil you will need.

Per serving (without lemon juice, using all oil): 71 calories; 7 grams fat; 1 gram protein; 2 grams carbohydrate

From Gigia

MARINATED SHIITAKE MUSHROOMS

Shiitake mushrooms provide trace minerals and are treasured by the Japanese and Chinese for their medicinal properties. Use these Japanese-style mushrooms as a garnish for rice, fish, chicken, or tofu.

Good for all three types.

Makes 4 servings

8 shiitake mushrooms	2 tablespoons tamari soy sauce
¼ cup water	2 tablespoons mirin (sweet Japanese
2 tablespoons honey	cooking wine)

Remove the mushroom stems and slice the caps into thin ribbons. Place them in a small saucepan and add the water, honey, and soy sauce. Simmer over medium-low heat until all the liquid has evaporated, stirring from time to time to keep the mushrooms from sticking to the pan. When the liquid has evaporated, add the mirin and roll the pan around to coat the mushrooms. Remove from the heat and cool to room temperature.

Per serving: 58 calories; 0 grams fat; 1 gram protein, 15 grams carbohydrate

From Gigia

ORANGE CHIPOTLE SALSA

This salsa is always an enormous hit. It requires so few ingredients and is so full of vibrant flavor that almost everyone loves it.

Chipotle chilies are ripe jalapeño peppers that have been dried and smoked. You can find them dried in packages or canned in adobo (a red chili sauce). The canned variety are easier to cook with and have a more complex flavor. This salsa is especially good with grilled shrimp or fish.

Wonderful for Vatas and Kaphas. Pittas might find the oranges too acidic and might also want to cut back on the amount of chilies called for in the recipe.

Makes 8 servings

6 navel oranges (preferably organic)	¼ cup fresh minced parsley
1 tablespoon chipotle chili in adobo, minced*	Pinch of salt, optional

Cut off the tops and bottoms of the oranges. Set each orange down on one of the cut sides and slice off the peel with a sharp knife. Cut the flesh in half and then into chunks.

Toss the orange chunks, chili, and parsley together. Taste, and add the salt if you wish.

Per serving: 53 calories; less than 1 gram of fat; 2 grams protein; 20 grams carbohydrate

* For a spicier salsa, add additional chilies.

From Indira

GREEN CHUTNEY

This might be a bit astringent for Vatas, who could combine it with rice and a protein for additional grounding. Pittas may want to cut down on the amount of chili in the recipe, or use a sweet green bell pepper instead.

Makes 10 servings

½ cup chopped cilantro
1 tablespoon peeled and chopped fresh
  ginger
1 tablespoon chopped fresh hot green
  chili
1 apple or avocado, peeled, seeded,
  and diced

2 tablespoons fresh lemon juice
½ teaspoon salt
Pinch of sugar (optional)
4 tablespoons water

Put all the ingredients in a blender and blend until smooth

Per serving (if using apple): 31 calories; 2 grams fat; 1 gram protein; 3 grams carbohydrate

From Gigia

MANGO SALSA

One serving of this nutrient-packed salsa gives you more than half your daily requirement of vitamin C and a third of your requirement for vitamin A. It's sweet and a good alternative to tomato-based salsa for those who like to spice up their food without adding a lot of heat. Try it in a bean burrito for a sweet surprise.

Good for all three types. Pittas might reduce the quantity of onion or even leave it out entirely.

Makes 8 servings

2 ripe but firm mangoes
½ red onion, chopped
½ red bell pepper, cored, seeded, and
   chopped in ¼-inch dice
1 tablespoon minced fresh ginger
¼ cup coarsely chopped fresh mint
   leaves

1 clove garlic, minced
Juice of 2 limes
Juice of ½ orange
1 jalapeño pepper, seeded and minced
1 teaspoon salt, or to taste

Peel the mangoes and cut the fruit off the center "bone." Dice the flesh into ¼-inch pieces.

Combine all the ingredients except the salt, taste, and add salt to taste.

Serve the salsa raw or warm it quickly to serve with chicken or fish.

Per serving: 42 calories; less than 1 gram fat; 1 gram protein; 10 grams carbohydrate

From Indira

RED CHUTNEY

This chutney is a bit heating, so it may be best for Vatas and Kaphas. Pittas might want to stick with the sweeter varieties of chutney. But it is really delicious!

Makes 10 servings

4 tablespoons oil
8 cloves garlic, coarsely chopped
4 small tomatoes, blanched and
   chopped
2 cups coarsely chopped onions

2 tablespoons paprika
6 tablespoons fresh lime juice
1 teaspoon sugar (optional)
Salt, to taste
Pinch of cayenne pepper

Heat the oil in a small skillet. Add the garlic and cook until it is soft. Stir in the tomatoes, then add the rest of the ingredients. Mix well and cook another 2 to 3 minutes. Cool briefly, then transfer the mixture to a blender and blend to a smooth paste.

Per serving: 75 calories; 6 grams fat; 1 gram protein; 6 grams carbohydrate

From Gigia

SWEET AND SPICY FRUIT CHUTNEY

Chutneys are relishes that let you customize your food to your own taste. This fruit chutney blends sweet and sour to make a fruit pickle. You can use whatever fruit is in season, including apples, pears, blueberries, or cranberries. Adjust the sweet and sour tastes to suit your own.

Vatas and Pittas might reduce the amount of garlic. The recipe is a bit heavy for Kaphas, but the heating, pungent spices can be helpful, so Kaphas might use this in small quantities.

Makes 12 servings

1½ cups unsulfured dried apricots	½ cup currants
1 cup pitted dates	1 cup turbinado sugar
2 cups hot water	¼ teaspoon salt
3 large cloves garlic	⅛ to ¾ teaspoon cayenne pepper
1 (2-inch) piece of fresh ginger	1 teaspoon ground cinnamon
½ cup red wine vinegar	½ teaspoon ground cloves
¾ cup raisins	½ teaspoon ground allspice

Soak the apricots and dates in 2 cups of hot water for 15 minutes, until they are soft. Drain the fruit, reserving the soaking liquid in case you need it later. Put the garlic, ginger, and ¼ cup of the vinegar into a food processor and blend until smooth. Add the apricots and dates and process until the fruit is coarsely chopped. The fruit should have a jamlike consistency; add a bit of the soaking liquid if it seems too dry.

Transfer the fruit mixture to a heavy stainless-steel or porcelain-lined pot and add the raisins and currants, the remaining vinegar, the sugar, salt, and spices. Bring the mixture to a boil, then simmer on medium heat, stirring frequently, for 20 minutes. Do not let the chutney stick to the bottom of the pot. Lower the heat if necessary, and cook until the fruit thickens and softens.

Taste, and adjust the flavors if necessary. While hot, the chutney will taste fairly sour, but it will sweeten as it cools. If it seems too thick, you can add some water. It will thicken slightly as it cools.

Cool at room temperature, then refrigerate in a lidded glass or ceramic bowl or jar. It will last indefinitely in the refrigerator.

Per serving: 180 calories; less than 1 gram fat; 2 grams protein; 47 grams carbohydrate

Desserts

To keep your taste buds happy and your body in balance, try to end each meal with a *small* sweet.

From Gigia

TOFU CHOCOLATE MOUSSE

For teenagers, or anyone who loves a chocolate indulgence, this is the dessert to have. In addition to containing soy protein, it's easier to make than traditional mousse because it requires no cooking. Real chocolate fiends should be sure to use good-quality cocoa powder and chocolate chips because you'll be satisfied with less. Make this for dessert and your friends will never know they're eating tofu.

Be careful how much of this you eat if digesting soy is a problem for you, and poor Kaphas should limit all their desserts. By eating the way we've been discussing, you might find out that all you need is a spoonful of something really nice in flavor anyway!

Makes 8 servings

½ cup chocolate chips
2 packages firm silken tofu
¼ cup unsweetened cocoa powder
½ cup maple syrup, or more to taste*

1 teaspoon vanilla extract
½ teaspoon salt
¼ cup Kahlúa or other liqueur of your
  choice

Melt the chocolate chips by heating them in the microwave for 30 seconds at a time on medium power. Stir after 30 seconds and repeat the process two or three times until they are melted to a smooth paste.

Combine all the ingredients, including the melted chocolate, in a blender and blend until smooth. Taste, and if you prefer a sweeter mousse add more maple syrup and blend again.

Spoon the mousse into individual serving cups or an attractive bowl and chill for 4 to 6 hours, until very cold.

Per serving: 195 calories; 7 grams fat; 7 grams protein; 27 grams carbohydrate

* If you prefer, you can use barley malt, rice syrup, or date sugar as a sweetener instead of the maple syrup.

Variation: You can make a fruit mousse using the same recipe but substituting pureed berries or mangoes in place of the chocolate chips and cocoa and a fruit liqueur instead of the Kahlúa.

From Gigia

RICE PUDDING

This is a traditional Indian and Ayurvedic sweet dessert that's wonderful for Vatas and Pittas. Kaphas might want to go easy—or enjoy a cup of chai with fresh fruit or a piece of crystallized ginger candy instead.

The flavors of cardamom, cinnamon, and rose water in this rice pudding add enough richness so that you won't miss the dairy. Rose water, a nonalcoholic flavoring made from rose petals and water, can be found in natural food stores as well as Middle Eastern and Indian markets. This also makes a great breakfast if served with some fresh fruit.

Makes 6 servings

1½ cups water
1 cup sweet rice*
1 teaspoon ground cardamom
1 teaspoon ground cinnamon
½ teaspoon ground black pepper
½ teaspoon salt

½ cup honey
2 cups almond milk
½ cup golden raisins
¼ cup blanched almonds, sliced or
   ground
2 teaspoons rose water (optional)

Bring the water to a boil in a heavy saucepan. Add the rice, cardamom, cinnamon, pepper, and salt. Cover the pan, turn the heat to low, and steam the rice for 20 minutes, until soft.

Remove the lid from the pot and add the honey, almond milk, raisins, and almonds. Stir until all the ingredients are well incorporated and heated through, about 5 minutes. Just before serving, stir in the rose water. Serve the pudding warm or cold.

Per serving: 208 calories; 2 grams fat; 3 grams protein; 46 grams carbohydrate

* Sweet rice is a short-grained glutinous rice also known as "sticky rice" in Thai cooking. It can be found in natural food stores and in Asian markets.

From Gigia

BAKED RICOTTA WITH BALSAMIC STRAWBERRIES

This light, fluffy, and simple tart is a good substitute for rich cheese-cake. The flavors of the spices and marinated strawberries more than make up for the richness of traditional cheesecake, and the ricotta and almonds provide good sources of protein.

Wonderful for Vatas, Pittas, and, in smaller quantities, Kaphas.

Makes 4 servings

For the Ricotta

½ cup blanched almonds
1 pound low-fat ricotta cheese
2 tablespoons honey

1 teaspoon cinnamon
1 teaspoon freshly grated orange
  zest

For the Strawberries

1 pint basket ripe strawberries
1 tablespoon balsamic vinegar

2 tablespoons maple syrup

Preheat the oven to 350 degrees.

Toast the almonds in the oven or in a dry pan for 8 minutes, then chop them fine or grind them in a food processor. Mix the almonds with the ricotta, honey, cinnamon, and orange zest. Spread the ricotta in an ungreased, 8-inch Pyrex pie pan to make a circle ½ inch thick.

Bake the ricotta in the preheated oven for 35 minutes, until the edges turn golden and the top is firm to the touch and beginning to turn pale brown.

While the ricotta bakes, rinse, stem, and slice the strawberries. Sprinkle them with the vinegar and toss them with the maple syrup. Let them marinate while the ricotta bakes and cools to room temperature. Cut the ricotta into wedges and spoon the strawberries on the side.

Per serving: 155 calories; 5 grams fat; 12 grams protein; 19 grams carbohydrate

Variations: Flavor the ricotta with lemon zest or brandy, and use walnuts, hazelnuts, or pine nuts instead of the almonds. Serve with whatever fruit is in season.

Beverages

From Indira

CHAI (Spiced Tea)

Makes 2 cups

2 cups water
¼ cup whole milk
1 to 2 teaspoons black tea
½ teaspoon chopped fresh ginger
2 pods cardamom, crushed

Pinch of black pepper
3 to 4 (½-inch-long) pieces fresh or
   dried lemongrass
Sugar, to taste (optional)

Bring the water, milk, tea, and spices (except the sugar) to a boil and boil for 2 to 3 minutes. Turn off the heat and steep the tea for 2 to 3 minutes. Strain and sweeten with sugar if you wish.

Per cup: 38 calories; 1 gram fat; 1 gram protein; 6 grams carbohydrate

For quick and easy chai: Instead of the spices in the recipe above, substitute the spices from one bag of Bengal Spice Celestial tea. Or you can buy premade chai from Yogi Teas or Oregon Chai. Add 2 ounces of almond, soy, rice, or whole milk, and drink warm or cool for a wonderful finish to any meal. It's warm and sweet, contains digestive spices, and can be as satisfying as a dessert. Many people find that it helps them cut down on their caffeine intake, and is a nice treat before bed if it is decaffeinated.

Vatas and Pittas should use decaf beverages and can use whole milk and a bit more sweetener. Kaphas should use almond or soy milk and more of the heating, pungent spices, such as cloves, cinnamon, and allspice.

From Jennifer

CCF TEA

This tea helps digestion for all three constitutional types. It cools Pitta, calms Vata, and reduces Kapha. Vatas and Pittas can add a drop of maple syrup to sweeten the tea.

Makes 1 serving

1 teaspoon coriander seed, lightly crushed

1 teaspoon fennel seed, lightly crushed

½ teaspoon cumin seed, lightly crushed

2 cups water

Bring all the ingredients to a boil and drink while hot—or drink cool in the summertime.

CHAPTER ELEVEN

A Final Word on How to Help Yourself and Make a Difference

If you've come this far, you may have figured out that I am devoted to the support of clean, organic, free-range food sources. I would recommend that you look into buying these products whenever possible, because I believe that this is one important way you can improve your own life and heath. The choices I personally make about the foods I eat, are based on my understanding of what will help to keep me healthy, happy, and balanced while also helping to preserve the health of our planet and the animals that live on it. I hope that after reading this chapter, you will want to learn even more.

I've spent the past five years researching organic, sustainable, and environmentally friendly food issues, and the more I learned, the more I came to realize how closely our health and our food system are interrelated. This book would not have been complete if I didn't take the opportunity to help you understand something of "the bigger picture" and the ways that the health and food delivery systems we've created may be impacting all our lives. I hope that once you have this information you might want to start supporting a more sustainable system of agriculture.

• • •

While there is no definitive proof of the correlation between the increase in particular health problems and the toxins in our food and environment, there's no doubt that certain types of problems are on the rise in this country.

Did you know that the American Cancer Society has predicted that approximately 182,000 women in this country will be diagnosed with invasive breast cancer in the next year? In March of 2000, Bill Moyers hosted a public television broadcast about environmental toxins and their potential effect on health. He quoted statistics to indicate that the rate of breast cancer in the United States has been rising steadily over the past four decades and that more than 40,000 women will die of the disease this year. The American Cancer Society estimates that 20 in every 100,000 American women develop breast cancer in their lifetime, while in China that number is 5 out of every 100,000, and in Japan it's 7 out of 100,000. According to a November 30, 1998, article in *Newsweek* magazine, Americans die of breast, prostate, and colon cancer at a rate that is five to thirty times higher than that of people in other parts of the world.

Sixteen out of every 100,000 American men develop prostate cancer, while in Japan that number is 5 out of every 100,000. More than 180,000 cases will be diagnosed in the next year, and approximately 32,000 men will die. Testicular cancer is also on the increase, and the number of diagnosed cases in young men between the ages of eighteen and thirty-two has risen more than 65 percent since 1972.

Given these statistics, it should be noted that the National Institutes of Health, which is funding research into the relationship between cancer and fruit and vegetable intake, has recommended that patients should get at least ten servings of fruits and vegetables each day. In addition, there is now ample evidence to suggest that fully 90 to 95 percent of all cancers are caused by environmental toxins and that, therefore, organic foods are very important for anyone who is trying to prevent, or recover from, cancer.

On that same Bill Moyers broadcast, Dr. Philip Landrigan, a pediatrician specializing in preventive medicine at the Mt. Sinai School of Medicine, stated that since 1972 we have experienced a 41 percent increase in the number of children diagnosed with brain cancer. Moreover, increasing numbers of children are being diagnosed with learning disabilities, and a recent article in *Mothering* magazine states that according to realistic estimates, there are approximately 5 million American school-age children currently being prescribed Ritalin. That number is up from 150,000 in 1970, between 250,000, and 541,000 in 1980, and 900,000 in 1990. The *Journal of the American Medical Association* estimates that Ritalin use in two-to-four-year-olds increased 200 percent to 300 percent between 1991 and 1995.

I quote these numbers not to frighten you, but simply to get you thinking. Most of us don't spend too much time looking at these problems until we or a loved one is diagnosed with a serious health problem. But it may be possible that simply changing the way we eat, exercise, and manage stress could prevent some of these conditions. The same *Newsweek* article mentioned above quoted a study conducted jointly by the World Cancer Research Fund and the American Institute for Cancer Research, which concluded that poor eating habits accounted for almost one-third of all cancers, almost the same number as is associated with smoking. As I said way back at the beginning of this book, we know what to do, so why are we not doing it? The Bill Moyers special also indicated that there are now more than 9,000 new *untested* chemicals on the market. While many chemicals have definitely made our lives better, there is also a possibility that many of these new chemicals are having effects on the health of the planet and our endocrine and hormonal systems.

I want to make it very clear that I do not deny the benefits of technology; I work with technology every day and couldn't run my life or my business without it. But I do believe there must be a way—and many researchers and experts in the field of organic and biodynamic farming have statistics to prove that there is—to take the best technology has to offer and to combine that knowledge with traditional agricultural practices to create a system that will benefit humans and at the same time be consciously kinder and gentler to the planet, the animals, and, ultimately, our children.

In 1992 Diane Dreher, author of *The Tao of Personal Leadership*, paid a visit to Shanghai, where she learned the water supply was so polluted that local residents couldn't drink it without boiling it first. The rapid rise of technology and industry had led to widespread pollution, particularly with respect to the drinking water. The lesson she draws from that is that when we are building our industrial base, we must not lose sight of our connection with the land, with natural cycles, and with the water, which is the source of all life.

John Jeavons, author of *How to Grow More Vegetables, Fruits, Nuts, Berries, Grains and Other Crops than You Ever Thought Possible on Less Land than You Can Imagine,* and an expert in the area of biointensive sustainable farming, has stated that biodynamic mini-farming is able to produce "two to six times the yield/unit area, and use 99 percent less energy, 50 to 100 percent less purchased nutrients, and 66 to 87 percent less water than conventional agricultural practices per pound of food produced." Our conventional farming methods are eroding farmable topsoil at an alarming rate. It would certainly seem that we're capable of doing better than we are now.

Throughout this book, I've emphasized the importance of recognizing and working with our own biological individuality, and it wouldn't make sense for me now to tell you that no one should ever again eat a dairy product, or a steak, or a chicken breast. But one of the main differences between the modern American diet and the diet of many other countries is the quantity of processed foods we eat in this country, along with our lack of physical activity and exercise. I believe that many of the diseases we suffer can be attributed not only to our lack of exercise, but also to our overconsumption of processed, nutrient-deficient foods. The irony is that these are foods *we have asked for* so that we can get more done in less time and hardly ever sit down to eat a quiet, peaceful family meal.

Because so many of us are Pitta personalities living in a perpetual Vata imbalance, we crave and ask for more and more heavy, grounding, creamy foods filled with sweet and salty tastes that can be eaten in a hurry. Those cravings just about sum up everything that fast-food chains with drive-through windows have to offer. Special sauces, pickles, and fries certainly provide the nurturing we seek. But at what price? The lack of quality and nutrients in those foods create the buildup of toxins in our bodies that lead to illness and obesity.

So how can we satisfy our cravings and still "make a difference" in the world? I believe it is through our support of organic, sustainable farming methods that not only produce food that tastes better and is more nutrient dense than foods treated with chemicals and hormones, but is also better for the land and more humane to animals.

It's just possible that by eating food that is more nutritious and satisfying, we would be able to better manage our weight, and then we might be able to reallocate some of the $50 billion we spend annually on weight loss to feed the hungry and educate the public about guarding the health of the land.

OVERWEIGHT AND UNDERNOURISHED

Despite the fact that some 55 percent of us, including approximately 11 million children, are overweight to obese, 10.5 million American households are experiencing some type of insecurity about where their next meal is coming from, and an estimated 14.4 million children living in those homes go to school and to bed hungry. This is happening in the United States.

I definitely do not believe that we have become so selfish that we're simply indifferent to the plight of these children. I choose to think that so many Americans are now so confused and overwhelmed by the volume of conflicting information they receive about health and nutrition that they simply don't have any energy left to devote to worrying about other people, our food delivery system, or the global picture. My hope for this book and The Balanced Approach is that by making it easier for you to manage your own health, I'll also be helping you to feel calmer and more nurtured, and that you then might be better able to think about the bigger picture, including environmental issues and the needs of the world's children and animals.

Anyone who's ever flown on a commercial airline has heard the flight attendant say that in case of emergency, you must put on your own oxygen mask first and then help your child or your neighbor. I hope that this book has helped you to gain a bit more understanding about your own body and given you a few more tools to nurture and care for yourself. If I can help you to do that for yourself, you might be able to spend just a little more time finding out how you can be part of the larger picture.

DISEASES OF ABUNDANCE

Personally, I've been blessed with the opportunity to work with some brilliant practitioners who have taught me an enormous amount and broadened my perspective tremendously.

One of these wonderful people is Dr. Sarita Shrestha, M.D., OB-GYN, the first female Ayurvedic physician in Nepal—no small feat—who now teaches advanced courses in Ayurveda each year at the Rocky Mountain Institute for Yoga and Ayurveda in Boulder, Colorado. Her insights into the differences between treating patients in Nepal and treating those in Los Angeles or Boulder are enlightening, if not necessarily surprising.

The biggest difference, she notes, is in the nature of the problems themselves. In Nepal, where most of the population is poor, the biggest health problem is malnutrition, along with gynecological problems resulting from a lack of education and health care facilities. But because of their understanding of Eastern philosophies and the concepts of karma and dharma, people there are more accepting of their place in the world and have a more spiritual outlook on life.

Americans, on the other hand, suffer more from emotional problems. Now that we have so many material things and so much technological advancement, we seem to be perpetually worried about losing what we have. We suffer from overwork and overworry. We spend too much time working and too little time with our families, and as a result, many of us are lonely, depressed, isolated, and sad. The amount of antidepressants used in the United States should be an indication that something is wrong.

In my own travels to countries like South Africa, Kenya, Egypt, Peru, and Ecuador, I too have seen a kind of poverty that we in America will never experience. And I have wondered why it is that, having so much, we are still suffering from so many illnesses associated with sadness, loneliness, and isolation.

I think that, on the one hand, America, like technology, has all the power and strength of a teenager or adolescent. What we don't have yet is the wisdom to best use that power and strength. We are suffering from an overabundance that is literally killing us, physically and emotionally. We are suffering from autoimmune diseases like chronic fatigue, fibromyalgia, multiple sclerosis, and lupus. Our bodies can't keep up the pace that we and technology have inflicted upon ourselves.

In a recent lecture, Paul Hawken, author of *The Ecology of Commerce,* founder of the Erewhon Trading company (a natural foods wholesaler), and one of the emerging leading philosophers of the sustainability movement, stated that "the 50 million people who will be added to the U.S. population over the next 40 years will have the same global impact in terms of using up resources as 2 billion people in India." We are blessed with so much in this country, yet our own prosperity would appear to be literally killing us and our planet.

AHIMSA, OR "CRUELTY FREE"

One of the aspects of Ayurveda that most appealed to me from the beginning was the theory of *ahimsa*, which means acting in a way that is nonviolent to other people and animals, as well as to ourselves and the planet.

The Bible tells us, "Do unto others as we would have them do unto us," while science tells us that $E = mc^2$, meaning that energy can be neither created nor destroyed, it just keeps changing form. Ayurveda believes that suffering is created by a lack of connection to "God or the universe," or to whatever version of that notion prevails in your particular belief system, and that the more disconnected we are from that primal source of energy, the more isolated and sad we will feel. And if there are children going hungry and animals living in terrible conditions, if our waters are polluted and our land is stripped of minerals just so that we can produce more food than we can ever eat in this country, then, I believe, we are suffering from that disconnection and actually feeling the pain we are inflicting on the planet. But what is the solution? How can we both feed the hungry and take care of the planet? If we eliminate world hunger, will we not create an overpopulation that would put even more stress on our natural resources?

FEEDING THE HUNGRY WHILE SAVING THE PLANET

A recent article by Joan Dye Gussow, Ph.D., Mary Swartz Rose Professor Emerita of Nutrition and Education at Teachers College, Columbia University, and author of *The Organic Life*, quotes Barbara Ward, co-founder and president of the International Institute for Environment and Development and another female pioneer in the field of sustainable development, on this very subject:

> It seems that birth rates have fallen, and we might still have a chance to feed the world's hungry without it being at the expense of

the planet and the animals. It would need to be done, however, with labor-intensive farming, meaning people working the land, research going into smaller farms instead of more tremendous, industrialized farms, and the use of solar energy on the farms, and recycling of organic material to reduce the need for pesticides, fertilizers, and use of weeding and insect control that makes use of people rather than chemicals.

These sorts of practices were current less than sixty years ago, right up until World War II. We now call it "organic" or "sustainable" agriculture and consider these methods impractical and inefficient— but it doesn't have to be that way. It is still possible to take the best of both worlds—traditional agriculture and industrialized agriculture— and create a sustainable agricultural model that would make the most of technology while still maintaining strict controls over the introduction of new, potentially harmful farming practices such as pesticides and genetically modified organisms. But it would take the commitment of all sides—the government, the corporations, and the consumers—working together for the health of humanity, the animals, and the planet. I believe we could do it if we wanted to.

When I asked Dr. Gussow recently what we could do to become more involved in making this come about, her answer was simply "to get more informed about and know where your food comes from." This may sound rather naive and oversimplified, but we've got to start somewhere. Why not simply try to get in touch with a local organic farmer and find out what it is he or she does? Then try to eat more fresh foods that are produced as close to your home as possible. Support your local farmers, and try to reduce the resources it takes to fly out-of-season food from across the country or halfway around the world. That's what the members of the Chefs Collaborative are trying to do.

I'm sure that by now you're familiar with the term *prana,* meaning vitality. The fresher the food, the more vitality and nutritional value it will have. And the same is true for our animals. Organic farmers support range-free, cage-free, pasture-fed livestock, who not only live better lives than those on large, industrial farms, but who also provide food that is healthier for us because they are healthier themselves. While we in the United States have not yet experienced the epidemics of hoof and mouth disease or mad cow disease that are ravaging the livestock in Great Britain, we can't be certain that these dreadful problems won't ever reach our shores. Personally, I can't help wondering whether the terrible conditions under which animals on industrial farms are forced to live, and the kinds of food and hormones they are being fed, aren't ultimately responsible for the diseases they fall prey to.

There are people who believe that the stress induced in animals that are kept penned and subjected to a variety of inhumane conditions on industrialized farms actually changes their hormonal profiles and lowers their immunity to disease. And from what we know about the ways that stress can impact the hormones of human beings who live in a fight-or-flight situation, this seems to me to be a logical conclusion to draw. Ayurveda, among other Eastern philosophies, believes that if we treat animals in this way, we will ingest the terrified, stressed, frightened energy of the animal, and this in turn will have a negative effect on our own health.

People Who Are Doing It

Theresa Murphy, M.S., R.D., is one person who is making the new organic/industrial paradigm work. She is chair of education and research for the Hunger and Malnutrition Dietetic Practice Group of the American Dietetic Association and currently works for the United Way in New York City.

She has obtained grants that allow the United Way in New York City to buy shares in a number of local community-supported agricultural farms in low-income areas of the city. These are organically run farms located all around the country, including in the boroughs of the Bronx, Brooklyn, and Queens in New York City, in which neighbors can buy shares and sometimes even work for their food. (When I joined one here in Boulder, we were able to feed three adults and two children over a period of six months for a total cost of $225, and we had so much produce left over that we were able to give some away.) The United Way then donates the food Theresa's shares have bought to emergency food shelters and food pantries for the hungry in the low-income neighborhoods where the farms are located. She also educates the recipients in becoming more self-sufficient and taking control of their own health by eating good, clean, nutritious food.

It's a win-win situation: the grant money helps to support local organic farmers, and low-income people get to eat good-quality, organic food and learn something about taking care of their own health. Since I'm from Queens and Manhattan, I was especially interested in Theresa's work. This is not just a "Boulder" phenomenon.

The Chefs Collaborative, some of whose members have graciously contributed recipes to this book, is another organization whose members are devoted to educating themselves and their customers about ways that we as individuals can have a positive impact on our food system and our health.

Founded in 1993, the Chefs Collaborative is a network of chefs, restaurateurs, and other culinary professionals who promote sustainable cuisine by teaching children, supporting local farmers, educating one another, and inspiring their customers to choose clean, healthy foods and "celebrate the pleasures of food." They describe themselves as people who "recognize the impact of food on our lives, on the well-being of our communities, and on the integrity of the environment. And who celebrate the joys of local, seasonal, sustainable cooking."

Whole Foods Market, founded in 1980 with one small store in Austin, Texas, is now the largest retailer of natural and organic foods, with 121 stores in 22 states and the District of Columbia. Whole Foods is dedicated to stringent quality goals and sustainable agriculture. Their Web site states that they "believe companies, like individuals, must assume their share of responsibility as tenants of planet Earth," and as Stephanie Solton, sales and marketing director for Whole Foods, Boulder, Colorado, told me when I spoke to her about this book, it is a company that truly "walks their talk." The company as a whole donates more than $2.4 million each year to charity, and individual local stores hold "CommUnity Days," when they donate a percentage of their sales to a nonprofit organization. They are proving that it is possible to be a "big business" and still take responsibility for preserving our precious natural resources. In fact, one of the benefits of shopping in a health food market such as Whole

Foods is that their employees are able to keep you informed about the latest developments in the food industry so that you can make an educated choice. I find their employees are well versed in the industry and happy to be working there. Whole Foods is obviously profitable and growing quickly and still interested in "the bigger picture."

The Earth Communications Office is another group I admire. It is a nonprofit, nonpartisan organization that "uses the power of communication to improve the global environment." With a board of directors, under Chairman Larry Kopald, comprising leaders in virtually all aspects of communication—from actors to musicians to film and theater professionals—the organization has created award-winning campaigns consisting of movie theater, television, and radio public announcements that have been seen in more than sixty-five countries worldwide.

Results International is another amazing group dedicated to ending world hunger through political activism and microcredits for small companies and individuals.

For other groups committed to ending world hunger and helping children and the environment, see pages 307–315.

MONEY TALKS

When it comes to determining the kinds of foods we want to have made available to us, we can make a difference simply by putting our money where our mouth is.

Statistics compiled by Datamonitor, a market research firm that tracks the organic industry, indicate that natural and organic foods constitute the fastest-growing segment of the retail food market and that sales have increased 20 percent in each of the past nine years.

If we build on those numbers by demanding more of these products on the retail level, we will not only contribute to lowering the prices of organic foods by encouraging an increase in volume, but we will prove to the agricultural industry and to the United States Department of Agriculture that it would be profitable to invest more dollars in support of organic farming. If we ask, long and loudly enough, we will be heard. But if we don't ask, we can't expect others to provide. One of the many advantages of living in a democratic, consumer-driven society is that we, as consumers, have the power to drive producers and suppliers to create the products we are willing to pay for.

Look for the words *Certified Organic* on the foods you buy. To receive certification from the Organic Trade Association, a farm must have been free of prohibited chemicals for a period of three years prior to certification, and the grower or processor must keep detailed records of his or her methods and materials, all of which must be inspected yearly by a third-party certifier. It takes a lot of work and dedication for companies, restaurants, and suppliers to comply with these standards, which is why I wanted to bring them to your attention, so that, knowing more about them, you might be more willing to lend your support.

I have found many companies that produce eggs from cage-free, free-range hens that have been given no hormones or antibiotics. I have found organic goat's milk products, cheese products, and wild fish. And I have found chicken, turkey, and beef farms that are organic and concerned about their animals as well as their customers.

And if spending is one effective way to help assure that we get what we want, keeping our wallets closed is another.

THE QUESTION OF GENETIC ENGINEERING

By now it would be virtually impossible for anyone who reads a newspaper or watches television news to be unaware of the fact that much of our food is being genetically engineered or modified. The intent, when these products were originally created, was to help put an end to world hunger, and no one is arguing that they should not be used to feed hungry people in impoverished countries. For various reasons involving patents and red tape, it seems these genetically engineered foods are simply not going to the places they were intended to serve. Instead, these products are appearing on our own grocery store shelves, and the important question being asked is, "Why are these foods not being labeled?" As Laura Ticcate, executive director of Mothers for Natural Law, put it to me:

> Here in the United States, the government allows GE [genetically engineered] foods on the market without thorough safety testing. Nor are they required to be labeled. Already over 60 percent of the foods on our grocery shelves contain some genetically engineered component—from infant formula to chips, pizza to ice cream, soda to burgers—and our kids are eating them every day.
>
> Are genetically engineered foods safe? No one knows. And in the meantime, our children have been turned into unwitting guinea pigs in the largest food experiment of all time. As a mother, I find this unconscionable.

Statistics published by the National Research Council indicate that more than seventy million acres of U.S. farmland are devoted to growing genetically modified crops. This includes more than half our soybean crop, one-third of our corn, and a large percentage of our cotton.

Given that we in America suffer from an overabundance rather than a lack of food, it's hard to understand why we need these products. And why, moreover, should we not be able to determine simply by reading a label whether or not a particular product is genetically engineered, so that we can decide for ourselves if we want to buy it? In fact, polls have shown that 70 to 80 percent of Americans do want genetically engineered products to be labeled. We would like to have a say in what we eat.

Some of you may think this isn't such a big deal, and for some of you, that may well be correct. If a product can be produced more economically through genetic engineering, and if it tastes good, and if you want to buy it, you should certainly be able to do that—assuming you know what you're buying.

But what about people who must be careful what they eat because they have a particular food allergy or sensitivity? Did you know, for example, that a fish gene has been added to certain tomatoes in order to lower their freezing temperature and preserve their freshness? What if you were allergic to fish, or simply chose not to eat fish because you were a vegetarian or because it was against your religious beliefs? Should you not be able to determine, when you go to the market, whether your tomato is still a tomato or whether it is now partly fish?

At the moment, the only way to be certain you are not eating genetically engineered foods is to buy organic.

One aspect of this reluctance to label is particularly interesting to me. Labeling is a marketing tool, and when producers or manufacturers know that we, the public, want something and are willing to pay for it, they are quick to advertise it loudly and clearly. This was proved in the last decade by the rush to label everything "lite," "reduced-fat," and "fat-free." "Cholesterol-free" is a popular label that is advertised even on nonanimal products such as peanut butter that never contained cholesterol in the first place! So I can only assume that if the manufacturers of these new foods really believed we wanted them and would buy them, they would be eager to let us know where to find them.

A FINAL WORD

I said at the beginning of this chapter that my food choices, and those I advocate, are about trying to keep myself and others healthy and well nourished while also nourishing our animals and our planet. But, where big business is concerned—and agriculture is certainly big business—politics also becomes involved, if only in the sense that we must make those in power understand what we want before we can expect to get it.

At heart I believe it is my job to bring some of these issues to your attention, because I do believe that by providing yourself with the freshest, cleanest, most nutritious, and tastiest food available, you will be protecting your own health and, ultimately, protecting the health of the world we live in.

I hope I have motivated you to learn a little more about the sources of the foods you eat, and I also hope that even if you don't agree with me, I have gotten you thinking. I hope you will still be able to use the information in the rest of this book to improve your health, remove some of the stress from your life, and better manage your weight.

Thank you for reading.

Aisle by Aisle: Buying What You'll Need

The following shopping list is not meant to be exhaustive or exclusionary. I couldn't possibly name every food or product you might need or want to buy. Nor do I expect that you'll never again come home with a loaf of rye bread or a container of Ben & Jerry's Chunky Monkey. I do, however, recommend that you try to buy organic whenever possible, and I try to recommend companies that produce clean products and operate in a way that is compassionate and "friendly" to animals and the environment.

My intention is to provide you with a guide to some of the basic foods and flavorings you may not have been familiar with or used before, so that when you try one of the recipes in this book, or when you prepare a familiar meal with a new twist for yourself and/or your family, you'll be able to reach into the cupboard or the refrigerator and find what you need.

Most of the items on this list can be found in local health food stores, and many conventional markets also now carry many of these products, but if you have difficulty finding any of them, please see page 299 or log on to our Web site at www.thebalancedapproach. com. for an explanation of some of these products.

PRODUCE

Plenty of fresh, organic fruits and vegetables, including dark leafy
greens such as kale, chard, and spinach, broccoli, bok choy (try
baby bok choy), mustard greens, and root vegetables like
squash, sweet potatoes, and yams. When you sauté them and
flavor them with a good chutney, you'll find that they are tastier
and more satisfying than you ever believed "healthy" vegetables
could be.

Again, the sweet, pungent taste from the chutney with the bitter
greens works really well.

You can buy frozen organic vegetables made by Cascadian Farms
or another purveyor of frozen organic vegetables.

DAIRY (AND NONDAIRY "DAIRY")/PROTEIN

These are complete proteins, too, for non–meat eaters.

Cheese*

Rice cheese, almond cheese, soy cheese (These are very good, high
in protein, and low in fat and cholesterol. They're great for
Kaphas, who have a sensitivity to dairy, but they do contain
trace amounts of casein, so be careful if you have an immediate,
IgE allergy to dairy.)

Goat cheese, which comes in various forms, including feta, herbed/
spiced goat cheese, and even sliceable Cheddar, Monterey Jack,
and mozzarella styles to serve with crackers

Cottage cheese

Other cheeses of your choice

1 or 2 ounces of cheese with 3 or 4 olives and a couple of Health Valley rice bran crackers makes a great snack.

* Many people think they need to give up cheese, but there are good substitutes out there that taste great.

Milk

Organic cow's milk
Almond milk
Soy milk
Rice milk

All of the above are fortified with vitamins A and D and calcium.

Yogurt

Goat's milk yogurt (Goat's milk is more heating and much less
    mucus-forming than cow's milk, which is homogenized and pas-
    teurized. It's great for kids or people who have congestion prob-
    lems.)
Soy yogurt
Stonyfield Farm organic yogurt

PROTEIN

See the list in chapter 3 for additional sources of protein. Remember
to rotate your sources of protein. Fish, for example, is healthy and
heart protective, on the one hand, but it can also contain excessive
amounts of mercury. According to the *Sustainable Seafood* report
put out by members of the Chefs Collaborative in collaboration with
the Environmental Protection Agency, pregnant women should not
eat tuna more than once or twice a week because of the mercury content.
    All organic and free-range whenever possible.

Eggs
Tofu
Fish
Chicken
Boca or Garden or Veggie Burgers (Great with rice or almond
    cheese and sautéed veggies.)
Fresh fish, especially wild, cold-water fish such as salmon, mack-
    erel, or tuna

Nuts and Seeds*

Nuts, such as almonds, walnuts, pine nuts, cashews, or soy nuts
Seeds, such as pumpkin, sunflower, or sesame

Bars and Shakes

ReBar organic fruit and vegetable bars (I love these. They're fairly
   high in carbohydrates, but their source is fruits and vegetables.)
Nutiva Nut and Hemp Bars

*Both of the above are organic and contain no genetically engineered
or modified organisms. They have a good ratio of protein to carbohydrates and good fats. They're both great for kids, and the Hemp Bars
are particularly good for people concerned with carbohydrate intake.
They contain no wheat, gluten, soy, or dairy.*

Balance Bars (in a pinch)
Luna Bars (These are higher in carbohydrates and are good for
   Vatas and endurance athletes.)

Protein Shakes

Metagenics Ultra Clear
Organic Prozone Rice Protein (vanilla flavored)
Spirutein, Peaceful Planet, or Solgar Soy Protein
Solgar Whey to Go

GRAINS AND STARCHES
(NONGLUTEN FOR SENSITIVITIES AND VARIETY)

Rice

Arborio (Italian)
Basmati (Indian)
Jasmine (Thai)
Brown

* They are not complete proteins but become so if mixed with grains or
beans and cheeses.

Fantastic and Lundgren make "quick" versions of the above that cook in 15 minutes.

Rice crust for pizza (Nature's Hilights)
Health Valley rice bran crackers (I love these as a snack with cheese or nut butter. Six crackers contain only 19 grams of carbohydrate, and you only need about 3 for a quick breakfast or a snack with some cheese or nut butter.)

Pastas and Grains

Quinoa
Corn/polenta
Buckwheat
Amaranth
Rice pasta
Lentil (bean), orso pasta (excellent for cold pasta salads with lots of vegetables), or other nongluten grains

Flours, Breads, and Bagels

Corn flour/cornmeal (masa harina)
Quinoa
Amaranth
Potato
Buckwheat
Glutino, gluten-free bagels and breads
Gluten-Free Pantry flours for cookies, breads, cakes, etc.
Wheat-free pancake and waffle mixes—usually made with potato, rice, or buckwheat flour
Food for Life rice/millet, rice/pecan, or rice/almond bread
Other nongluten grains

Hot Cereals

Don't forget to add cinnamon and cardamom and a drop of maple syrup, and eat your cereal with some protein.

Quinoa
Rice
Corn
Amaranth

Millet
Buckwheat/kasha
Other nongluten grains

CANNED GOODS

Bearito's Organic

Refried beans (Wonderful for quick burritos with corn tortillas, vegetables, salsa, and guacamole.)
Pinto beans
Black beans

Health Valley Soups

These are tasty and lower in sodium than regular canned soups. Great for kids or when you get home late and are tired. Remember to add good spice, additional vegetables, and 2 to 3 ounces of cheese for additional protein and grounding.

14 Garden Vegetable
Tomato Vegetable
Lentil
Black bean
Chicken and Rice
Split pea

Tuna (Dolphin-Safe)

For a quick and easy lunch, I love this tuna with 1 tablespoon of canola mayonnaise, 1 teaspoon of mango chutney, 1 slice of rice cheese, 2 to 3 Salsa Mesquite Kettle Potato Chips, and 1 to 2 cups of vegetables, with herbs and spices like curry or garam masala. Add a cup of soup and you have something warm, protein, and vegetables with herbs and spices, and good oils.

OILS AND SPREADS

Try to buy organic whenever possible.

Oils

Extra-virgin olive oil
Canola
Walnut
Sesame
Ghee (organic clarified butter)

Spreads

Almond butter
Peanut butter
Tahini
Cashew butter
Macadamia nut butter
All-fruit preserves (such as Cascadian Farms or Sorrell Ridge) with
   no sugar added (These are really sweet, even without additional
   sugar or corn syrup.)

SWEETS, SWEETENERS, AND SNACKS

Many of these sweets are actually very low in carbohydrates because
there is no sugar added. They are good quality and have vibrant
taste, so you should only need a little.

Sweeteners

Maple syrup
Honey
Sucanat
Cane sugar
Date sugar

Chocolate

A little piece of good-quality chocolate goes a long way.

Ghirardelli Sweet Cocoa
Ahlaska chocolate or any organic cocoa powder

Check the label: 1 teaspoon of cocoa powder, as opposed to syrups with added sugar, is under 3 grams of carbs—very satisfying as a snack in the evening with some warm milk or in a protein shake.

Dagoba or other organic chocolate

Dagoba does a great job of blending organic chocolate with spices like cinnamon, ginger, chai, chilies, and lime.

Snacks

Terra Chips or other natural nonhydrogenated chips
Organic nuts, such as almonds, cashews, walnuts, etc.
Organic dried fruits, such as dates, raisins, apricots, etc. (all non-sulfured)

A cup of soup with 1 to 2 ounces of organic nuts and/or seeds or cheese and ½ piece of fresh fruit or a few pieces of dried fruit makes a great snack.

Stretch Island Fruit Leather Roll Up snacks (Great for kids and adults with a sweet tooth. Has 12 grams of carbohydrate in a whole Roll Up.)
Sharkies Totally Natural Sports Snacks (Electrolyte replacement fruit snacks. Great for kids and athletes. Has 2 to 3 grams of carbohydrate per piece.)
Planet Harmony organic fruit bear snacks and fruit snacks (Kids love these—adults, too. Has 2 to 3 grams of carbohydrate per piece.)
Pamela's Rice Cookies (wheat and gluten free)
Crystallized ginger candy
Edamame beans (These are fresh Japanese soybeans—they're full of protein, very low on the glycemic index, and a good, salty protein snack. You can buy them already cooked or frozen in many markets.)

These sweet treats are all fruit and very low in sugar and carbohydrates.

Herbs, Spices, and Flavorings

Check the shelves in your local health food store. There are many great spice blends, chutneys, and salsas that will add flavor and life to your food with very few additional calories or carbs.

Indian flavorings such as Patak's Major Grey's Chutney, mango lime chutney, or hot chutney, mild curry, muchi curry, and others

Wheat-free tamari or ginger tamari

Thai flavors/spaces, including peanut satay sauce, green curries, red curries, and peanut coconut sauces. Thai Kitchen is one of my favorite brands.

Mexican spices of your choice, such as salsas, guacamole, or picante sauces

Japanese flavorings such as wasabi and fresh or pickled ginger

African blends from Collection Africa, such as Sweet Zambezi Sauce, Zulu Open Fire Sauce, and Voodoo Hot Sauce

Dried

Look for organic. Try Frontier or Simply Organic blends and singles. The ones I usually suggest clients try first are garam masala, curry, Mexican spice blend, and Italian/Mediterranean spice blend. Also:

Anise

Cardamom

Cinnamon

Coriander

Cumin

Fennel

Flaxseeds (grind and use 1 tablespoon in coffee)

Herbs de Provence (A French blend of rosemary, thyme, sage, and lavender.)

Tofu Scramble (Fantastic Foods)

Turmeric

Other herbs and spices of your choice. Let your nose be your guide. Just start experimenting by adding ¼ to ½ teaspoon to soups or sautéed vegetables.

Salt

Sea salt
Orsa salt
Celtic sea salt

BEVERAGES

Teas

Green tea
Peppermint
Chamomile
Vata, Pitta, Kapha teas
Be Trim tea
Grandma's Tummy Mint
Eater's Digest
PMS
CCF (cumin, coriander, and fennel; see page 263)

Juices

For children, in particular, it's important that these be organic. Try Mountain Sun Knudsen's Organic with no added sugar (these are sweet and satisfying all by themselves):

Apple
Cranberry
Grape

SUPPLEMENTS

EFAs

Fish oils: Omega 3's (EPA/DHA): Metagenics, Country Life
Essential Fatty Acid Blends (vegetarian in liquid form): Spectrum, Twin Lab, Udo's Choice
Total EFAs by Health from the Sun (contains flaxseed oil, borage oil, evening primrose oil, and lecithin)
Wild Alaskan salmon oil: Natural Factors

Flaxseed oil or ground flaxseeds (vegetarian source)
Hemp seed oil: Nutiva

Liquid Amino Acids:

Bragg's

Probiotics

Metagenics Ultra Flora (dairy free) or PB8, Natural Factors, Jarrow, and New Chapter (There are different strains for children, adults, and seniors—ask in your local health food store.)

Green Foods

Solgar Greens and More powder or pills or Nutri-greens (or similar green food blends) include spirulina, alfalfa, barley greens, and other greens.

NONFOOD ITEMS

Soft-bristled dry brush for the skin (Earth Therapeutics makes a nice soft one.)
Body oils such as sesame oil, grape seed oil, almond oil, coconut oil
Essential oils: lavender, sandalwood, lemon, grapefruit, eucalyptus, etc. (Look for Young Living Oils, a therapeutic-grade oil of excellent quality that is available through many complementary practitioners such as massage therapists and nutritionists.)

APPENDIX B

The Glycemic Index

Food	Glycemic Index
Bakery Products	
Cake, sponge	460
Cake, banana, made with sugar	47
Cake, pound	54
Cake, banana, made without sugar	55
Pastry	59
Pizza, cheese	60
Muffins	62
Cake, flan	65
Cake, angelfood	67
Croissant	67
Crumpet	69
Doughnut	76
Waffles	76
Beverages	
Soy milk	30
Cordial, orange	66
Soft drink, Fanta	68

Food	Glycemic Index
Breads	
Barley kernel bread	39
Rye kernel bread	46
Fruit loaf	47
Oat bran bread	48
Mixed-grain bread	48
Pumpernickel	50
Bulgur bread	53
Linseed rye bread	55
Pita bread, white	57
Hamburger bun	61
Rye flour bread	64
Semolina bread	64
Oat kernel bread	65
Barley flour bread	67
Wheat bread, high-fiber	68
Wheat bread, wholemeal flour	69
Melba toast	70
Wheat bread, white	71
Bagel, white	72
Kaiser rolls	73
Whole-wheat snack bread	74
Bread stuffing	74
Wheat bread, Wonderwhite	78
Wheat bread, gluten free	90
French baguette	95
Breakfast Cereals	
Rice Bran	19
Kellogg's All Bran Fruit 'n Oats	39
Kellogg's Guardian	41
All-Bran	42
Porridge (oatmeal)	49
Red River Cereal	49
Bran Buds	53
Special K	54
Oat Bran	55
Kellogg's Honey Smacks	55
Muesli	56
Kellogg's Mini-Wheats (whole wheat)	57
Bran Chex	58
Kellogg's Just Right	59
Life	66

Food	Glycemic Index

Breakfast Cereals (continued)

Food	Glycemic Index
Nutri-grain	66
Grape-Nuts	67
Sustain	68
Shredded Wheat	69
Kellogg's Mini-Wheats (blackcurrant)	69
Cream of Wheat	70
Wheat Biscuit	70
Golden Grahams	71
Pro Stars	71
Sultana Bran	71
Puffed Wheat	74
Cheerios	74
Corn Bran	75
Breakfast bar	76
Total	76
Cocoa Pops	77
Post Flakes	80
Rice Krispies	82
Team	82
Corn Chex	83
Cornflakes	83
Crispix	87
Rice Chex	89
Rice Bubbles	90

Cereal Grains

Food	Glycemic Index
Barley, pearled	25
Rye	34
Wheat kernels	41
Rice, instant, boiled, 1 min.	46
Bulgur	48
Rice, parboiled	48
Rice, parboiled, high amylose	48
Barley, cracked	50
Wheat, quick cooking	54
Buckwheat	55
Sweet corn	55
Rice, specialty	55
Rice, brown	55
Rice, wild, Saskatchewan	57
Rice, white	58
Rice, white, high amylose	58

Food	Glycemic Index
Cereal Grains (continued)	
Cous-cous	65
Barley, rolled	66
ice, Mahatma Premium	66
Taco shells	68
Cornmeal	69
Millet	71
Rice, Pelde	76
Rice, Sunbrown Quick	80
Tapioca, boiled with milk	81
Rice, Calrose	87
Rice, parboiled, low amylose Pelde	87
Rice, white, low amylose	88
Rice, instant, boiled 6 min.	90
Cookies	
Oatmeal cookies	55
Rich Tea cookies	55
Digestives	59
Shredded Wheatmeal	62
Shortbread	64
Arrowroot	67
Graham Wafers	74
Vanilla Wafers	77
Morning Coffee cookies	79
Crackers	
Jatz	55
High Fibre Rye Crispbread	65
Breton Wheat Crackers	67
Stoned Wheat Thins	67
Sao	70
Water Crackers	71
Rice Cakes	77
Puffed Crispbread	81
Dairy Foods	
Yogurt, low-fat, artificially sweetened	14
Milk, chocolate, artificially sweetened	24
Milk + 30 g. bran	27
Milk, full fat	27
Milk, skim	32
Yogurt, low-fat, fruit sugar sweetened	33

Food	Glycemic Index
Dairy Foods (continued)	
Milk, chocolate, sugar sweetened	34
Yogurt, unspecified	36
Milk + custard + starch + sugar	43
Yakult (fermented milk)	45
Ice cream, low-fat	50
Ice cream	61
Fruit and Fruit Products	
Cherries	22
Grapefruit	25
Apricots, dried	31
Pear, fresh	37
Apple	38
Plum	39
Apple juice	41
Peach, fresh	42
Orange	44
Pear, canned	44
Grapes	46
Pineapple juice	46
Peach, canned	47
Grapefruit juice	48
Orange juice	52
Kiwi fruit	53
Banana	54
Fruit cocktail	55
Mango	56
Sultanas	56
Apricot, fresh	57
Pawpaw	58
Apricot, canned, syrup	64
Raisins	64
Rockmelon (muskmelon, cantaloupe)	65
Pineapple	66
Watermelon	72
Legumes	
Soybeans, canned	14
Soybeans	18
Lentils, red	25
Beans, dried, not specified	28
Lentils, not specified	29

Food	Glycemic Index
Legumes (continued)	
Kidney beans	29
Lentils, green	29
Butter beans + 5 g. sucrose	30
Butter beans + 10 g. sucrose	31
Butter beans	31
Split peas, yellow, boiled	32
Lima beans, baby, frozen	32
Chick peas (garbanzo beans)	33
Kidney beans, autoclaved	34
Haricot/navy beans	38
Pinto beans	39
Chick peas, curry, canned	41
Black-eyed beans	41
Chick peas, canned	42
Pinto beans, canned	45
Romano beans	46
Baked beans, canned	48
Kidney beans, canned	52
Lentils, green, canned	52
Butter beans + 15 g. sucrose	54
Beans, dried, *P. Vulgaris*	70
Broad beans (fava beans, foul moudammas)	79
Pasta	
Spaghetti, protein enriched	27
Fettuccine	32
Vermicelli	35
Spaghetti, wholemeal	37
Star pastina	38
Ravioli, durum, meat filled	39
Spaghetti, boiled 5 min.	36
Spaghetti, white	41
Spirali, durum	43
Capellini	45
Macaroni	45
Linguine	46
Instant noodles	47
Tortellini, cheese	50
Spaghetti, durum	55
Macaroni and cheese	64
Gnocchi	67
Rice pasta, brown	92

Food	Glycemic Index
Vegetables	
Peas, dried	22
Peas, green	48
Sweet corn	55
Pumpkin	75
Broccoli	0–15
Kale	0–15
Collards	0–15
Bok choy	0–15
Spinach	0–15
Lettuce	0–15
Root Vegetables	
Yam	51
Sweet potato	54
Potato, white, not specified, boiled	56
Potato, new	57
Potato, white, Ontario	60
Potato, canned	61
Potato, Prince Edward Island, boiled	63
Beets	64
Potato, steamed	65
Potato mashed	70
Carrots	49
Swede (rutabaga)	72
Potato, boiled, mashed	73
French fries	75
Potato, microwaved	82
Potato, instant	83
Potato, baked	85
Parsnips	97
Snack Food and Confectionary	
Peanuts	15
Mars M&M's (peanut)	32
Mars Snickers Bar	40
Mars Twix Cookie Bars (caramel)	43
Mars Chocolate (Dove)	44
Jams and marmalades	49
Chocolate	49
Potato chips	54
Popcorn	55
Muesli bars	61

Food	Glycemic Index
Snack Food and Confectionary (continued)	
Mars Kudos Whole Grain Bars (choc. chip)	61
Mars Bar	64
Mars Skittles	69
Life Savers	70
Corn chips	74
Jelly beans	80
Pretzels	81
Dates	103
Soups	
Tomato soup	38
Lentil soup, canned	44
Split pea soup	60
Black bean soup	64
Green pea soup, canned	66
Sugars	
Fructose	22
Lactose	46
Honey	58
High-fructose corn syrup	62
Sucrose	64
Glucose	96
Glucose tablets	102
Maltodextrin	105
Maltose	105

Resource Guide

ORGANIC FOOD COMPANIES

Ahlaska Certified Organic Cocoa
www.ahlaska.com
800-431-4018

Annie's Naturals
www.annienatural.com
800-434-1234

Coleman Natural Beef
www.colemanmeats.com
800-442-8666

Earth Harvest Foods (nut butters)
www.earthharvestfoods.com
604-222-3015

Hains/Health Valley/Celestial Seasonings/Terra Chips
www.hain-celestial.com
516-237-6200

Hempola
www.hempola.com
800-240-9215

Horizon Organic Dairy, Inc.
www.horizonorganic.com
303-530-2711

Lundberg Family Farms
www.lundberg.com
530-882-4551

Newman's Own
www.newmansownorganics.com
408-685-2866

Organic Valley
www.organicvalley.com
608-625-2602

Pacific Foods of Oregon, Inc.
www.pacificfoods.com
503-692-9666

Rice Slice cheese
Soyco Foods
Orlando, FL
www.galaxyfoods.com
800-808-2325

Small Planet Food/Cascadian Farm (now owned by General Mills)
 (organic frozen vegetables, etc.)
www.smallplanetfoods.com
513-474-9773

Solana Gold Organics and Appleseed Farms
800-459-1121

Stonyfield Farm
www.stonyfield.com
603-437-4040

V Bar Beef, LLP
719-783-2461

Whole Foods
www.wholefoods.com

Wild Oats
www.wildoats.com

ETHNIC FLAVORS, SPICES, DRESSINGS, CONDIMENTS

Annie Chun's Inc.
www.anniechun.com
415-479-8272

Collection Africa Exotic Food
Natural Group, Inc.
www.printempsgourmet.com
209-522-6860

Frontier Natural Products
www.frontiercoop.com
303-449-8137

Home Grown Natural Foods
www.consorzio.com
707-254-3700

Melissa's
www.melissas.com
800-468-7111

Patak's Original (chutneys)
800-726-3648

San-J International, Inc. (tamaris, soy sauces, marinades)
www.san-j.com
800-446-5500

Seeds of Change
www.seedsofchange.com
323-586-4853

Sorrell Ridge/Allied OLD English, Inc.
www.sorrellridge.com
800-225-0122

Tasty Bite
Preferred Brands Inc.
www.tastybite.com
203-698-4041

Thai Kitchen
www.thaikitchen.com
510-268-0209

SNACKS, BARS, AND SWEETS FOR KIDS AND ADULTS

Dagoba Chocolate
www.dagobachocolate.com
303-473-9632

Endangered Species Chocolate Company
www.chocolatebar.com
541-535-2170

Fiji Ginger Company
www.fijiginger.com
310-452-0878

Imagine Foods
www.imaginefoods.com
650-595-6336

The Jewel Date Co.
760-399-4474

Kettle Foods (chips)
www.kettlefoods.com
503-364-0399

Nutiva (organic bars, hemp products)
www.nutiva.com
707-823-2800

Oasis Date Gardens
www.oasisdate.com
800-827-8017

Pamela's Products, Inc.
www.pamelasproducts.com
541-552-9520

Planet Harmony Organic Fruit Snacks
Harmony Foods Corporation
www.harmonyfoods.com
831-457-3370

ReBar Organic Food Bars
Healthco Canada Enterprises, Inc.
www.healthcocanada.com
250-868-5716

Rella Good Cheese Co.
www.rella.com
512-282-3110

Sharkies
www.sharkade.com
303-499-9073

Stretch Island Fruit, Inc. (fruit leather)
www.stretch-island.com
800-863-7836

WHEAT FREE/GLUTEN FREE

Adrienne's Gourmet Foods
www.adriennes.com
805-964-6848

Food for Life Baking Co., Inc.
www.food-for-life.com
800-797-5090

The Gluten-Free Pantry
www.glutenfree.com
860-633-3826

Glutino (bagels, breads)
www.glutino.com
800-363-3438

Nature's Hilights (pizza crust)
916-342-6154

Pamela's Products, Inc.
www.pamelasproducts.com
541-552-9520

Quinoa Corporation
www.quinoa.net
310-530-8666

Seeds of Change
www.seedsofchange.com
323-586-4853

Van's International Foods
Christine A. Kempe
www.vansintl.com
310-320-8611

BEVERAGES

Ahlaska Certified Organic Cocoa
www.ahlaska.com
800-431-4018

Celestial Seasonings
www.celestialseasonings.com
800-351-8175

Golden Temple, Sunshine and Yogi Tea
www.goldentemple.com
800-225-3623

Mountain Sun
www.mountainsun.com
636-462-4741

Naked Juice
www.nakedjuice.com

Odwalla (juices)
www.odwalla.com
800-odwalla

Oregon Chai
www.sellchai.com
888-874-2424

Santa Cruz Organic Juices/Knudsen
www.knudsenjuices.com
530-899-5000

Teeccino (coffee substitute)
www.teeccino.com
805-966-0999

Traditional Medicinal (teas)
www.traditionalmedicinal.com
707-823-8911

EARTH-FRIENDLY CLEANING PRODUCTS

Into Balance
www.intobalance.com
888-345-4686

Seventh Generation
www.seventhgen.com
802-658-3773

SUPPLEMENTS

For more information about some of these products and companies, please check our Web site (www.thebalancedapproach.com) under the "Products" button.

Champion Nutrition
www.champion-nutrition.com
800-225-4831

Country Life
www.country-life.com
800-645-5768

Maharishi Ayur-Veda
www.mapi.com
800-255-8332

Mega Food
www.megafood.com
773-263-8940

Metagenics
www.metagenics.com
800-692-9400

Naturade, Inc.
www.naturade.com
800-421-1830

Nature's Formulary
www.naturesformulary.com
800-923-9338

New Chapter
www.new-chapter.com
800-543-7279

Planetary Formulas
www.planetaryformulas.com

Solgar
www.solgar.com
800-645-2246

Young Living Essential Oils (aromatherapy)
See www.thebalancedapproach.com

ENVIRONMENTAL/SUSTAINABLE/SAFE FOOD COMPANIES

Bioneers
www.bioneers.org
877-246-6337

The Center for Food Safety
www.foodsafetynow.org
202-547-9359

Chefs Collaborative
www.chefnet.com/cc2000
781-736-0635

Citizens for Health
www.citizens.org
303-417-0772

ECO—Earth Communications Office
www.OneEarth.org
310-656-0577

Ecofish
www.ecofish.com
603-269-5555

Environmental Working Group
www.ewg.org
202-667-6982

Greenpeace
www.greenpeace.org

The Land Institute
www.landinstitute.org
785-823-5376

Mothers and Others for a Livable Planet
www.mothers.org
212-242-0010

Mothers for Natural Law
www.safe-food.org
641-472-2499

National Organic Directory
www.caff.org/caff/publications/nod_1997.html
800-852-3832

Organic Trade Association
www.ota.com
413-774-7511

Oldways Preservation and Exchange Trust
www.oldwayspt.org

SOCIAL CONSCIOUSNESS

Global Renaissance Alliance
www.renaissancealliance.org
202-544-1219

Institute for Global Communications (IGC)
www.igc.org

John Jeavons
Bountiful Gardens
Ecology Action
Willits, CA
www.bountifulgardens.org
707-459-6410

LOHAS Journal
www.lohasjournal.com
303-442-8983

RESULTS
www.results.action.org
202-783-7100

YOGA

Yoga Alliance
www.yogaalliance.com
877-964-2255

Yoga International
www.yimag.org

Yoga Journal
www.yogajournal.com

Yoga: Living Arts:
www.livingarts.com
800-2Living

Ayurvedic Centers

Alandi Ashram and Ayurvedic Gurukula
Boulder, CO
303-786-7437

The Ayurvedic Institute and Wellness
  Center
Dr. Vasant Lad
Albuquerque, NM
www.ayurveda.com
505-291-9698

Chopra Center for Well Being
La Jolla, CA
www.chopra.com
619-551-7788

John Douillard
Boulder, CO
www.lifespa.com
303-516-4848

The Himalayan Institute
Honesdale, PA
www.himalayaninstitute.org
800-822-4547

Maharishi Ayur-Veda
Colorado Springs, CO
www.mapi.com
800-826-8424

National Ayurvedic Medical Association (NAMA)
www.ayurveda-nama.org
info@ayurveda-nama.org
800-292-4882

National Institute of Ayurvedic Medicine
NYC, NY
Dr. Scott Gerson, M.D.
www.niam.com
212-505-8971

The Rocky Mountain Institute of Yoga and Ayurveda
Boulder, CO
Sarasvati Buhrman, Ph.D.
Pat Hansen, M.S.
www.earthnet.net/rmiya
303-443-6923

Dr. Dennis Thompson, D.C.
Rejuvenation
Boulder, CO
303-417-0941

MEDICAL

American Celiac Society
59 Crystal Ave.
West Orange, NJ 07051
973-325-8837
www.stepstn.cono/nord/org_sum/1270.htm

American Holistic Health Association
www.ahha.org
714-779-6152

American Holistic Medical Association
McLean, VA
www.holisticmedicine.org
703-556-9728

Celiac Disease Foundation
13251 Ventura Blvd., Suite 1
Studio City, CA 91604
818-990-2354
www.celiac.org/cdf

Crohn's and Colitis Foundation of America, Inc.
386 Park Avenue South, 17th fl.
New York, NY 10016-7374
800-932-2423 or 212-685-3440

Gluten Intolerance Group of North America
15110 10th Ave., SW, Suite A
Seattle, WA 98166-1820
206-246-6652

Health Equations (nutritional blood testing)
Dr. Lynne August, M.D.
Newfane, VT
www.healtheqs.com
802-365-9213

Institute for Functional Medicine
Dr. Jeffrey Bland, Ph.D.
www.fxmed.com
800-228-0622

FITNESS

American Council on Exercise
San Diego, CA
www.acefitness.org
858-535-8227

C.h.e.k. Institute
www.paulchekseminars.com
800-552-8789

Deportes International
New York, NY
Ben Velàzquez
917-553-8670

Inside Out Fitness
Billy Corbett
Denver, CO
303-378-1488

International Sports Sciences Association (ISSA)
Santa Barbara, CA
www.issa-usa.com
800-892-ISS

Medical Fitness Services
Denver, CO
Glenn Streeter
303-528-6729

National Fitness Therapy Association
Winter Park, CO
www.nfta.org
970-726-0697

Poliquin Performance Center
Tempe, AZ
Charles Poliquin
www.charlespoliquin.net
480-966-3840

PILATES

Balanced Body
www.pilates.com
800-745-2837

Body Dynamics
Integrated Health and Fitness Specialists
Boulder, CO
303-440-5776

Jennifer Kries
www.peterpan.com
201-344-4214

Bobbie Nigro
Pilates at World Gym
Rego Park, NY
718-464-6382
718-459-3248

Moira Stott-Merrithew
www.stottpilates.com
800-910-0001

The Pilates Center
www.thepilatescenter.com
303-494-3400

The Pilates Studio at Drago's Gym
New York, NY
212-757-0724

CHILDREN/HUNGER

Children International
www.children.org
800-888-3089

Feed the Children
800-627-4556

The Hunger Site
www.thehungersite.com

RESULTS
results.action.org
202-783-7100

Save the Children
www.savethechildren.org

Unicef
www.unicefusa.org
212-686-5522

ANIMAL AWARENESS

All for Animals
www.allforanimals.com

www.animalconcerns.netforchange.com
www.arrs.envirolink.org

Animal Protection Institute
www.api4animals.org

PETA
www.peta-online.org

Political Voice for Animals
www.pva@pva-colorado.org

APPENDIX D

Further Reading

INTRODUCTION

Bruinsma, K., and Taren, D. L. Chocolate: Food or drug? *Journal of the American Dietetic Association,* 99, 10 (1999): 1249–56.

Daush, Judy. Determining when obesity is a disease. *Journal of the American Dietetic Association,* 101, 3 (2001): 293.

Duffy, V., and Bartoshuk, L. Food acceptance and genetic variation in taste. *Journal of the American Dietetic Association,* 100, 6 (2000): 647–55.

Duffy, V., Fast, K., Cohen, Z., and Bartoshuk, L. Genetic taste status associates with fat food acceptance and body mass index in adults. *Chemical Senses,* 24 (1999): 545–46.

Glanz, K., Milbach, B., and Goldberg, S. Why Americans eat what they do: Taste, nutrition, cost, convenience, and weight control concerns as influences on food consumption. *Journal of the American Dietetic Association,* 98 (1998): 1118–26.

Hill, A. J., and Heaton-Brown, L. The experience of food craving: A prospective investigation in healthy women. *Journal of Psychosomatic Research,* 38, 8 (1994): 801–14.

Kanarek, R. B., Ryu, M., and Przypek, J. Preference for foods with varying levels of salt and fat differ as a function of dietary restraint and exercise but not menstrual cycle. *Physiology and Behavior,* 57 (1995): 821–26.

Papkin, B., and Doak, C. The obesity epidemic is a worldwide phenomenon. *Nutrition Reviews,* 56, 4 (1998): 106–14.

Patel, Vimal. Ayurveda: Science of integrative approaches to health and disease. *International Journal of Integrative Medicine,* 1, 5 (1999): 7–9.

Senekal, M., Albertse, E. C., Momberg, D. J., Groenewald, C. J., et al. A multidimensional weight-management program for women. *Journal of the American Dietetic Association,* 99, 10 (1999): 1257–63.

Simopoulos, A. P. Genetic variants, diet, and physical activity. *Journal of the American Dietetic Association,* 101, 3 (2001): 302–04.

CHAPTER ONE

Chopra, Deepak. *Perfect Health.* New York: Random House, 1991.

Douillard, John. *Body, Mind and Sport.* New York: Crown Publishers, 1995.

Frawley, David. *Yoga and Ayurveda.* Twin Lakes, Wisc.: Lotus Press, 1999.

———. *Ayurveda and the Mind.* Twin Lakes, Wisc.: Lotus Press, 1996.

Johari, Harish. *The Healing Cuisine*. Rochester, Vt.: Healing Arts Press, 1994.

Lad, Vasant. *Ayurveda: The Science of Self-Healing*. Twin Lakes, Wisc.: Lotus Press, 1984.

———. *The Complete Book of Ayurvedic Home Remedies*. New York: Random House, 1998.

Lad, Vasant and Frawley, David. *The Yoga of Herbs*. Twin Lakes, Wisc.: Lotus Press, 1986.

Morningstar, Amadea. *Ayurvedic Cooking for Westerners*. Twin Lakes, Wisc.: Lotus Press, 1995.

Thompson, Dennis. *Ayurvedic Zone Diet*. Twin Lakes, Wisc.: Lotus Press, 1999.

Tierra, Michael. *Planetary Herbology*. Twin Lakes, Wisc.: Lotus Press, 1988.

Tirtha, Swami Sada Shiva. *The Ayurveda Encyclopedia*. Bayville, N.Y.: Ayurvedic Holistic Center Press, 1998.

CHAPTER THREE

Anderson, J. V., Bybee, D. I., Brown, R. M., McLean, D. F., et al. 5 a day fruit and vegetable intervention improves consumption in a low income population. *Journal of the American Dietetic Association,* 101 (2001): 195–202.

Associated Press. Hormone may be key to diabetes. *New York Times,* Jan. 18, 2001.

Atkins, Robert C. *Dr. Atkins' Diet Revolution*. New York: Bantam Books, 1972.

Atkins, Robert C., and Gare, Fran. *Dr. Atkins' New Diet Revolution.* New York: M. Evans and Co, 1994.

Bang, H. O., Dyerberg, J., and Sinclair, H. M. The composition of the Eskimo food in north western Greenland. *American Journal of Clinical Nutrition.* 33, 12 (1980): 2657–61.

Belluzzi, A., Brignola, C., Campieri, M., Pera, A., Boschi, S., and Miglioli, M. Effect of an enteric-coated fish-oil preparation on relapses in Crohn's disease. *The New England Journal of Medicine,* 334, 24 (1996): 1557–60.

Block, G., Patterson, B., and Subar, A. Fruit, vegetables, and cancer prevention: A review of the epidemiological evidence. *Nutrition and Cancer,* 18, 1 (1992): 1–29. Review.

Broekmans, W. M., Klopping-Ketelaars, L.A., Schuurman, C. R., Verhagen, H., et al. Fruits and vegetables increase plasma carotenoids and vitamins and decrease homocysteine in humans. *Journal of Nutrition,* 130, 6 (June 2000): 1578–83.

Bronsgeest-Schoute, H. C., van Gent, C. M., Luten, J. B., and Ruiter, A. The effect of various intakes of omega 3 fatty acids on the blood lipid composition in healthy human subjects. *American Journal of Clinical Nutrition.* 34, 9 (1981): 1752–57.

Burgess, J. R., Stevens, L., Zhang, W., and Peck, L. Long-chain polyunsaturated fatty acids in children with attention-deficit hyperactivity disorder. *The American Journal of Clinical Nutrition,* 71, 1 (2000): 327–30.

Chidley, E. AHA dietary guidelines: What's new? *Today's Dietitian,* Feb. 01, 2001: 40–41.

Cyclical dieting poses dangers. *Medical World News,* Nov. 14, 1988: 25.

D'Adamo, Peter J., and Whitney, Catherine. *Eat Right for Your Type.* New York: G. P. Putnam's Sons, 1996.

DiPasquale, Mauro. *The Anabolic Diet*. Ontario, Canada: Optimum Training Systems, 1995.

Donahue, R. R., Abbott, R. D., Bloom, E., Reed, D. M., and Yano, K. Central obesity and coronary heart disease in men. *Lancet*, 1, 8537 (1987): 821–24.

Douillard, John. *The Three Season Diet*. New York: Harmony Books/Random House, 2000.

Ducimetiere, P., Richard, J., and Cambien, F. The pattern of subcutaneous fat distribution in middle-aged men and the risk of coronary heart disease: The Paris prospective study. *International Journal of Obesity*, 10, 3 (1986): 229–40.

Eades, Michael R., and Eades, Mary Dan. *Protein Power*. New York: Bantam Books, 1996.

Erasmus, Udo. *Fats That Heal, Fats That Kill*. Burnaby, B.C., Canada: Alive Books, 1986.

Farquhar, J. W., Frank, A., Gross, R. C., and Reaven, G. M. Glucose, insulin, and triglyceride responses to high and low carbohydrate diets in man. *Journal of Clinical Investigation*, 45 (1996): 1648–56.

Fritsch, J. "95% Regain Lost Weight. Or Do They?", *New York Times* (Health and Fitness section), May 25, 1999.

Kidd, P. M. Attention deficit/hyperactivity disorder (ADHD) in children. Rationale for its integrative management. *Alternative Medicine Review*, 5, 5 (2000): 402–28.

Leson, Gero, Pless, Petra, and Roulac, John W. *Hemp Foods & Oils for Health*. Sebastopol, Calif.: Hemptech, 1999.

Leventhal, L. J., Boyce, E. G., and Zurier, R. B. Treatment of rheumatoid arthritis with gammalinolenic acid. *Annals of Internal Medicine*, 119 (9): 867–73.

————. Treatment of rheumatoid arthritis with black currant seed. *British Journal of Rheumatism,* 33 (1994): 847.

London, S. J., Yuan, J. M., Chung, F. L., et al. Isothiocyanates, glutathione S-transferase M1 and T1 polymorphisms, and lung-cancer risk: A prospective study of men in Shanghai, China. *Lancet,* 356 (2000): 724–29.

McKeon, N. Antioxidants and breast cancer. *Nutrition Review,* 57 (1999): 321–24.

National Institutes of Health. Technology Assessment Conference on Obesity, 1992.

Nestle, M. Broccoli sprouts in cancer prevention. *Nutrition Review,* 56 (1998): 127–30.

O'Keefe, J. H., and Harris, W. S. From intuit to implementation: Omega-3 fatty acids come of age. *Mayo Clinic Proceedings,* 75, 6 (2000): 607–14.

Ornish, Dean. *Eat More, Weigh Less.* New York: HarperCollins, 1993.

Reaven, G. M. The role of insulin resistance and hyperinsulinemia in coronary heart disease. *Metabolism,* 41, 5 (Suppl. 1) (1992): 16–19.

————. Banting lecture, 1988. Role of insulin resistance in human disease. *Diabetes,* 37, 12 (1988): 1595–1607.

Richardson, A. J., and Puri, B. K. The potential role of fatty acids in attention-deficit/hyperactivity disorder. *Prostaglandins, Leukotrienes, Essential Fatty Acids,* 63, 1–2 (2000): 79–87.

Schmid, Ronald F. *Native Nutrition.* Rochester, Vt.: Healing Arts Press, 1987.

Sears, Barry. *Mastering the Zone.* New York: Regan Books/HarperCollins, 1997.

Sears, Barry, and Lawrence, Bill. *The Zone.* New York: Harper-Collins, 1995.

Shapiro, Laura. Is fat that bad? *Newsweek,* April 21, 1997: 59–64.

Simopoulos, A. P. Omega-3 fatty acids in health and disease and in growth and development. *American Journal of Clinical Nutrition,* 54, 3 (1991): 438–63.

Smith, D. L., Willis, A. L., Nguyen, N., Conner, D., Zahedi, S., and Fulks, J. Eskimo plasma constituents, dihomo-gamma-linolenic acid, eicosapentaenoic acid and docosahexaenoic acid inhibit the release of atherogenic mitogens. *Lipids,* 24, 1 (1989): 70–75.

Steward, Leighton H., Bethea, Morrison, C., Andrews, Sam S., and Balart, Luis A. *Sugar Busters!.* New York:Ballantine Books, 1998.

Stoll, A. L., Severus, W. E., Freeman, M. P., Rueter, S., Zboyan, H. A., Diamond, E., Cress, K. K., and Marangell, L. B. Omega 3 fatty acids in bipolar disorder. *Archives of General Psychiatry,* 56 (1999): 407–412.

Thompson, B., Demark-Wahnefried, W., Taylor, G., McClelland, J. W., et al. Baseline fruit and vegetable intake among adults in seven 5 A Day study centers in diverse geographic areas. *Journal of the American Dietetic Association,* 99 (1999): 1241–1248.

Thompson, Dennis. *Ayurvedic Zone Diet.* Twin Lakes, Wisc.: Lotus Press, 1999.

What's new at the FDA: Informing consumers about *trans* fat labeling. *Journal of the American Dietetic Association,* 100, 10 (2000): 1132.

Zurier, R., Jacobson, et al. Gamma-linolenic acid treatment of rheumatoid arthritis. *Arthritis & Rheumatism,* 39, 11 (1996): 1808–17.

CHAPTER FOUR

Alexander, J. A., Hunt, L. W., and Patel, A. M. Prevalence, pathophysiology, and treatment of patients with asthma and gastroesophageal reflux disease. *Mayo Clinic Proceedings,* 75, 10 (Oct. 2000): 1055–63.

Bucco, Gloria. New York, new hope. *Natural BusinessCommunications/Lohas Journal,* May/June 2000: 23–24.

Dajani, E. Z. Gastroesophageal reflux disease: Pathophysiology and pharmacology overview. *Journal of Academic Minority Physicians,* 11, 1 (2000): 7–11.

Eisenberg, D. M., Davis, R. B., Elmer, S. L., Appel, S., et al. Trends in alternative medicine use in the United States, 1990–1997: Results of a follow-up national survey. *Journal of the American Medical Association,* 280, 18 (Nov. 11, 1998): 1569–75.

Frawley, David. *Yoga and Ayurveda.* Twin Lakes, Wisc.: Lotus Press, 1999.

Lad, Vasant. Causative factors of ama. *Ayurveda Today,* 12, 2 (2000): 1–4.

Maron, P. N., and Burton, M. E. Antacids revisited: A review of their clinical pharmacology and recommended therapeutic use. *Drugs,* 57, 6 (June 1999): 855–70.

Pert, Candace. *Molecules of Emotion.* New York: Touchstone/Simon & Schuster, 1997.

Vanloon, G. Feeding agni. *Yoga International,* April/May 1998: 66–68.

Chapter Five

Balch, James F. and Balch, Phyllis A. *Prescription for Nutritional Healing*. Garden City Park, N.Y.: Avery Publishing Group, 1997.

Belluzzi, A., Boschi, S., Brignola, C., Munarini, A., et al. Polyunsaturated fatty acids and inflammatory bowel disease. *American Journal of Clinical Nutrition*. 71, suppl. (2000): 339S–342S.

Bland, Jeffrey S., Costarella, Linda, Levin, Buck, Liska, DeAnn, et al. *Clinical Nutrition: A Functional Approach*. Gig Harbor, Wash.: Institute for Functional Medicine, 1999.

Braly, James. *Dr. Braly's Food Allergy & Nutrition Revolution*. New Caanan, Conn.: Keats Publishing, Inc., 1992.

Carini, C., Brostoff, J., and Wraith, D. G. IgE complexes in food allergy. *Annals of Allergy*, 59, 2 (Aug. 1987): 110–17.

Coburn, Jennifer. Breastfeeding. *Mothering*, July/August 2000: 60–68.

Collins, M. D., and Gibson, G. R. Probiotics, prebiotics and symbiotics: Approaches for modulating the microbial ecology of the gut. *American Journal of Clinical Nutrition*, 69, 5 (1999): 1052S–1057S.

D'Adamo, Peter J., and Whitney, Catherine. *Eat Right for Your Type*. New York: G. P. Putnam's Sons, 1996.

Davis, M. K., Savitz, D. A., and Graubard, B. I. Infant feeding and childhood cancer. *Lancet*, 2, 8607 (Aug. 1988): 365–68.

Egger, J., Carter, C. M., Wilson, J., Turner, M. W., and Soothill, J. F. Is migraine food allergy?: A double-blind controlled trial of oligoantigenic diet treatment. *Lancet*, 2, 8355 (1983): 865–69.

Fisher, J. O., Birch, L. L., Smiciklas-Wright, H., and Picciano, M. F. Breast-feeding through the first year predicts maternal control in feeding and subsequent toddler energy intakes. *Journal of the American Dietetic Association*, 100 (2000): 641–46.

Gorbach, S. L. Probiotics and gastrointestinal health. *American Journal of Gastroenterology,* 95, suppl. (Jan. 2000): S2–S4.

Hadijivassiliou, M., Grunewalk, R. A., and Davies-Jones, G. A. B. Gluten sensitivity: A many-headed hydra. *British Medical Journal,* 318, 7200 (June 1999): 1710–11.

Halpern, G. M., and Scott, J. R. Non-IgE antibody mediated mechanisms in food allergy. *Annals of Allergy,* 58, 1 (Jan. 1987): 14–27. Review.

Hunter, J. O. Food allergy—or enterometabolic disorder? *Lancet,* 338, 8765 (Aug. 1991): 495–96.

Kidd, P. M. Attention deficit/hyperactivity disorder (ADHD) in children: Rationale for its integrative management. *Alternative Medicine Review,* 5, 5 (2000): 402–28.

Kopp-Hoolihan, Lori. Prophylactic and therapeutic uses of probiotics: A review. *Journal of the American Dietetic Association,* 101 (2001): 229–38, 241.

Lad, Vasant. Ojas. *Ayurveda Today,* spring 1995: 3–7.

Lanting, C. I., Fidler, V., Huisman, M., Touwen, B. C. L., and Boersma, E. R. Neurological differences between 9-year-old children fed breast milk or formula-milk as babies. *Lancet,* A344, 1994: 1319–22.

Macfarlane, G. T., and Cummings, H. Probiotics and prebiotics: Can regulating the activities of intestinal bacteria benefit health? *British Medical Journal,* 318 (1999): 999–1003.

Nettleton, J. A. Are Ω-3 fatty acids essential nutrients for fetal and infant development? *Journal of the American Dietetic Association,* 93, 1 (1993): 58–64.

Nsouli, T. M., Nsouli, S. M., Linde, R. E., O'Mara, F., et al. Role of food allergy in serious otitis media. *Annals of Allergy,* 73, 3 (1994): 215–19.

Rector-Page, Linda G. *Healthy Healing: An Alternative Healing Reference*. Healthy Healing Publications, 1985/1992.

Sampson, H. A., and Burks, A. W. Mechanisms of food allergy. *Annual Review of Nutrition*, 16 (1996): 161–77.

Schmid, Ronald F. *Native Nutrition*. Rochester, Vt.: Healing Arts Press, 1987.

Shu, X. O., Linet, M. S., Steinbuch, M., Wen, W. Q., et al. Breast-feeding and risk of childhood acute leukemia. *Journal of the National Cancer Institute*, 91, 20 (Oct. 20, 1999): 1765–72.

Simopoulos, A. P. Omega-3 fatty acids in health and disease and in growth and development. *American Journal of Clinical Nutrition*, 54, 3 (1991): 438–63.

Solderholm, J. D., Peterson, K. H., Olaison, G., Franzen, L. E., et al. Epithelial permeability to proteins in the noninflamed ileum of Crohn's disease. *Gastroenterology*, 117, 1 (1999): 65–72.

Weil, Andrew. *8 Weeks to Optimum Health*. New York: Fawcett Columbine/Ballantine Publishing Group, 1997.

Wolcott, William L., and Fahey, Trish. *The Metabolic Typing Diet*. New York: Doubleday/Random House. 2000.

Wyatt, J., Vogelsang, H., Hubl, W., Waldhoer, T., and Lochs, H. Intestinal permeability and the prediction of relapse in Crohn's disease. *Lancet*, 341, 8858 (June 5, 1993): 1437–39.

CHAPTER SIX

Allison, D. B., Fontaine, K. R., Manson, J. E., Stevens, J., and Van-Itallie, T. B. Annual deaths attributable to obesity in the United States. *Journal of the American Medical Association*, 282, 16 (Oct. 27, 1999): 1530–38.

American College of Sports Medicine (ed.). *Guidelines for Exercise Testing and Prescription,* 3rd. ed. Philadelphia: Lea & Febiger, 1986.

Blair, S. N. Evidence for success of exercise in weight loss and control. *Annals of Internal Medicine,* 119, 7 pt. 2 (1993): 702–6.

Borzekowski, D. L., and Robinson, T. N. The 30-second effect: An experiment revealing the impact of television commercials on food preferences of preschoolers. *Journal of the American Dietetic Association,* 101, 1 (2001): 42–46.

Colgan, Michael. *Optimum Sports Nutrition: Your Competitive Edge.* New York: Advanced Research Press, 1993.

Cope, Stephen. *Yoga and the Quest for the True Self.* New York: Bantam Books, 2000.

Dausch, Judy. Determining when obesity is disease. *Journal of the American Dietetic Association,* 101, 3 (2001): 293.

DiPasquale, Mauro. *The Anabolic Diet.* Ontario, Canada: Optimum Training Systems, 1995.

Epstein, L. H., Wing, R. R., and Valoski, A. Childhood obesity. *Pediatric Clinics of North America,* 32, 2 (1985): 363–79.

Gastelu, Daniel, and Hatfield, Fred. *Dynamic Nutrition for Maximum Performance.* Garden City Park, N.Y.: Avery Publishing Group, 1997.

Grodstein, F., Levine, R., Troy, L., Spencer, T., et al. Three-year follow-up of participants in a commercial weight loss program: Can you keep it off? *Archives of Internal Medicine,* 156, 12 (1996): 1302–6.

Hatfield, Frederick C., ed. *Fitness: The Complete Guide.* Santa Barbara, Calif.: International Sports Sciences Association, 1996.

Lee, Bruce. *The Tao of Jeet Kune Do.* Santa Clarita, Calif.: Ohara Publications, Inc., 1975.

Ornish, D., Brown, S. E., Scherwitz, L. W., Billings, J. H., et al. Can lifestyle changes reverse coronary heart disease?: The lifestyle heart trial. *Lancet,* 336, 8708 (1990): 129–33.

Poliquin, Charles. *Modern Trends in Strength Training: Volume 1* (2nd ed.). Napa, Calif.: Dayton Writers Group, 1997.

———. *The Poliquin Principles.* Napa, Calif.: Dayton Writers Group, 1997.

Rector-Page, Linda G. *Healthy Healing: An Alternative Healing Reference.* Healthy Healing Publications, 1985/1992.

CHAPTER EIGHT

Abuzakouk, M., and O'Farrelly, C. Diet, fasting, and rheumatoid arthritis. *Lancet,* 339, 8784 (Jan. 4, 1992): 68.

Berkowsky, Bruce. Skin brushing, rejuvenation, circulation & vital chi. *Massage & Bodywork,* October/November 2000: 12–20.

Haas, Elson M. *A Diet for all Seasons.* Berkeley, Calif.: Celestial Arts, 1981.

Jensen, Bernard. *Dr. Jensen's Juice Therapy.* Chicago: NTC/Contemporary Publishing Group, 2000.

Kjeldsen-Kragh, J., Mellbye, O. J., Haugen, M., Mollnes, T. E., et al. Changes in laboratory variables in rheumatoid arthritis patients during a trial of fasting and one-year vegetarian diet. *Scandinavian Journal of Rheumatology,* 24, 2 (1995): 85–93.

Percival, M. Nutritional support for detoxification. *Applied Nutritional Science Reports,* 1997: NUT023.

Serure, Pamela. *Three Days to Vitality.* New York: HarperCollins Publishers, 1997.

CHAPTER NINE

Agarwal, A. K., Singh, M., Gupta, N., Saxena, R., et al. Management of giardiasis by an immuno-modulatory herbal drug Pippali rasayana. *Journal of Ethnopharmacology,* 44, 3 (Dec. 1994): 143–46.

Ahmad, N., and Mukhtar, H. Green tea polyphenols and cancer: Biologic mechanisms and practical implications. *Nutrition Review,* 57, 3 (March 1999): 78–83.

Ammon, H. P., Safayhi, H., Mack, T., and Sabieraj, J. Mechanism of anti-inflammatory actions of curcumine and boswellic acids. *Journal of Ethnopharmacology,* 38, 2–3 (March 1993): 113–19.

Azuine, M. A., and Bhide, S. V. Chemopreventive effect of turmeric against stomach and skin tumors induced by chemical carcinogens in Swiss mice. *Nutrition and Cancer,* 17, 1 (1992): 77–83.

Balch, Phyllis A., and Balch, James F. *Prescription for Nutritional Healing.* Garden City, N.Y.: Avery Publishing Group, 2000.

Baskaran, K., Kizar Ahamath, B., Radha Shanmugasundaram, K., and Shanmugasundaram, E. R. Antidiabetic effect of a leaf extract from Gymnema sylvestre in non-insulin-dependent diabetes mellitus patients. *Journal of Ethnopharmacology,* 30, 3 (Oct. 1990): 295–300.

Bowtell, J. L., Gelly, K., Jackman, M. L., Patel, A., et al. Effect of oral glutamine on whole body carbohydrate storage during recovery from exhaustive exercise. *Journal of Applied Physiology,* 86, 6 (June 1999): 1770–77.

Chan, M. M., Ho, C. T., and Huang, H. I. Effects of three dietary phytochemicals from tea, rosemary and turmeric on inflammation-induced nitrite production. *Cancer Letter,* 96, 1 (Sept. 4, 1995): 23–29.

Colgan, Michael. *Optimum Sports Nutrition: Your Competitive Edge.* New York: Advanced Research Press, 1993.

Frawley, David, and Lad, Vasant. *The Yoga of Herbs.* Twin Lakes, Wisc.: Lotus Press, 1986.

Hadady, Letha. *Asian Health Secrets.* New York: Three Rivers Press, 1996.

Hatfield, Frederick C. (ed.) *Fitness: the Complete Guide.* Santa Barbara, Calif.: International Sports Sciences Association, 1996.

Heinerman, John. *The Complete Book of Spices.* New Canaan, Conn.: Keats Publishing, Inc., 1983.

Lowery, L. M., Appicelli, P. A., and Lemon, P. W. R. Conjugated linolenic acid enhances muscle size and strength gains in novice bodybuilders. *Medical Science of Sports and Exercise,* 30 (1998): S182.

Madsen, H., and Bertelsen, G. Spices as antioxidants. *Trends in Food Science Technologies,* 6, 1995 (1995): 271–77.

Mishra, L.-C., Singh, B. B., and Dagenais, S. Scientific basis for the therapeutic use of *Withania somnifera* (Ashwagandha): A review. *Alternative Medicine Review,* 5, 4 (2000): 334–46.

Scalzo, Richard, and Cronin, Michael. *Herbal Solutions for Healthy Living.* Brevard, N.C.: Herbal Research Publications, 2001.

Schulick, Paul. *Ginger: Common Spice and Wonder Drug.* Brattleboro, Vt.: Herbal Free Press, 1994.

Shanmugasundaram, E. R., Rajeswari, G., Baskaran, K., Rajesh Kumar, B. R., et al. Use of Gymnema sylvestre leaf extract in the control of blood glucose in insulin-dependent diabetes mellitus. *Journal of Ethnopharmacology,* 30, 3 (Oct. 1990): 281–94.

Tadi, P. P., Teel, R. W., and Lau, B. H. Organosulfur compounds of garlic modulate mutagenesis, metabolism, and DNA binding of aflatoxin B1. *Nutrition and Cancer*, 15, 2 (1991): 87–95.

Tierra, Michael. *Planetary Herbology.* Twin Lakes, Wisc.: Lotus Press, 1988.

Van der Hulst, R. R., van Kreel, B. K., von Meyenfeldt, M. F., Brummer, R. J. et al. Glutamine and the preservation of gut integrity. *Lancet*, 341, 8857 (1993): 1363–1365.

Chapter Ten

Fenster, Carol. *Special Diet Solutions.* Littleton, Colo.: Savory Palate, Inc., 1997.

Hagman, Bette. *The Gluten-free Gourmet Cooks Fast and Healthy.* New York: Henry Holt, 1996.

Johari, Harish. *The Healing Cuisine, India's Art of Ayurvedic Cooking.* Rochester, Vt.: Healing Arts Press, 1994.

Lad, Usha, and Lad, Vasant. *Ayurvedic Cooking for Self-Healing.* Albuquerque, N. Mex.: The Ayurvedic Press, 1994.

Morningstar, Amadea. *Ayurvedic Cooking for Westerners.* Twin Lakes, Wisc.: Lotus Press, 1995.

Morningstar, Amadea, and Desai, Urmila. *The Ayurvedic Cookbook.* Twin Lakes, Wisc.: Lotus Press, 1990.

McDermott, Nancie. *Real Vegetarian Thai.* San Francisco: Chronicle Books, 1997.

CHAPTER ELEVEN

Block, G., Patterson, B., and Subar, A. Fruit, vegetables, and cancer prevention: A review of the epidemiological evidence. *Nutrition and Cancer,* 18, 1 (1992): 1–29.

Cowley, G. Cancer & diet. *Newsweek,* Nov. 30, 1998: 60–66.

Crow, David. *In Search of the Medicine Buddha: A Himalayan Journey.* New York: Jeremy P. Tarcher/Putnam, 2000.

Gussow, J. D. *This Organic Life: Confessions of a Suburban Homesteader.* White River Junction, VT: Chelsea Green Publishing Co., 2001.

———. Will we destroy the environment trying to grow food for everyone?. *Kids Can Make a Difference Newsletter,* 6, 1 (2001): 3–4.

Marcotte, L. P. Food security in the United States: What's going on?. *Hunger Line: A Publication of the American Dietetic Association Hunger & Malnutrition Dietetic Practice Group,* 2000: 1.

Robbins, John. *Diet for a New America.* Walpole, N.H.: Stillpoint, 1987.

———. *May All Be Fed: Diet for a New America.* New York: Avon Books, 1992.

Index